CRITICAL CARE FINALS

FINALS

SAQs, EMQs and MCQs

Edited by

PHILIP STATHER
MBChB MRCS
Core Surgical Trainee 2, Northampton General Hospital, UK

and

HELEN CHESHIRE
MBChB DRCOG
GP Registrar, East Midlands South Deanery, UK

Radcliffe Publishing
London • New York

Radcliffe Publishing Ltd
33–41 Dallington Street
London
EC1V 0BB
United Kingdom

www.radcliffepublishing.com

British Library Cataloguing in Publication Data

A catalogue record for this book is available from the British Library.

ISBN-13: 978 184619 558 7

The paper used for the text pages of this book is FSC® certified. FSC (The Forest Stewardship Council®) is an international network to promote responsible management of the world's forests.

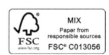

MIX
Paper from
responsible sources
FSC
www.fsc.org   FSC® C013056

Typeset by Phoenix Photosetting, Chatham, Kent, UK
Printed and bound by TJI Digital, Padstow, Cornwall, UK

Contents

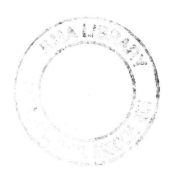

Acknowledgement

I dedicate this book to my wife; without her love, support and understanding this book would not have been possible.

Preface

This book aims to be a complete guide to passing your surgical finals. It is the only book containing SAQs, EMQs and MCQs, covering all surgical specialties. With over 140 SAQs, 65 EMQs and 130 MCQs with explanatory answers we hope that this text enables thorough preparation for exams, and improves your problem-solving skills through its variety of questions.

Please note that this is intended as a revision book, and we would refer you to other textbooks for continued learning.

We hope you find this a useful tool for your revision, and wish you the best of luck in your career.

Mr P Stather and Dr H Cheshire
September 2011

About the Editors

Philip Stather graduated from Leicester Medical School in 2007. He is currently working as a core surgical trainee in the East Midlands South Deanery.

Helen Cheshire graduated from Leicester Medical School in 2007. She is currently working as a GP registrar in the East Midlands South Deanery.

Contributors

Dr Saba Ahmed MBChB BSc
FY1 Kettering General Hospital

Dr Scott Castell MBChB
FY1 Kettering General Hospital

Dr Laura Dalton MBChB
FY1 Kettering General Hospital

Dr Nicholas Eastley MBChB
Core Surgical Trainee 1, Kettering General Hospital

Dr Wai Kien Ng MBChB
FY1 Kettering General Hospital

Dr Gita S Patel MBChB
FY2 Kettering General Hospital

Mr Alexander Rawlinson BSc MBChB MRCS(Ed)
Core Surgical Trainee 1, Northampton General Hospital

Dr Georgina Riddiough MBChB (Hons)
FY1 Northampton General Hospital

Dr Shafiq Arif Shahban BSc MBChB
FY1 Kettering General Hospital

Dr Pandora Spillman-Henham MBBS BSc (Hons)
FY1 Kettering General Hospital

Mr Philip Stather MBChB MRCS
Core Surgical Trainee 2, Northampton General Hospital

Abbreviations

AAA	abdominal aortic aneurysm
ABPI	ankle brachial pressure index
ACTH	adrenocorticotrophic hormone
AF	atrial fibrillation
AFP	alphafetoprotein
AIDS	acquired immunodeficiency syndrome
AP	antero posterior
APTT	activated partial thromboplastin time
ASA	American Society of Anesthesiology
AST	aspartate transaminase
ATLS	acute trauma life support
BMI	body mass index
BPH	benign prostatic hypertension
BPPV	benign paroxysmal positional vertigo
BRCA	breast cancer
Ca	calcium
CABG	coronary artery bypass graft
CBD	common bile duct
CLO	campylobacter-like organism test for *H. pylori*
CMV	cytomegalovirus
CNS	central nervous system
CPAP	continuous positive airway pressure
CRP	C-reactive protease
CSF	cerebrospinal fluid
CTS	carpal tunnel syndrome
DDH	developmental dysplasia of the hips
DVT	deep vein thrombosis
EBV	Epstein Barr virus
ERCP	endoscopic retrograde cholangiopancreatography
ESR	erythrocyte sedimentation rate
FAST	focused assessment sonography in trauma

FBC	full blood count
FESS	functional endoscopic sinus surgery
FNAC	fine needle aspiration cytology
FSH	follicle stimulating hormone
GA	general anaesthetic
GCS	Glasgow Coma Score
GI	gastrointestinal
GIT	gastrointestinal tract
GORD	gastroesophageal reflux disease
GTN	glycerine tri-nitrate
HCC	hepatocellular carcinoma
HIV	human immunodeficiency virus
ICP	intracranial pressure
IHD	ischaemic heart disease
IV	intravenous
IVDU	intravenous drug user
JVP	jugular venous pressure
KUB	kidneys, ureters, bladder
LA	local anaesthetic
LDH	lactate dehydrogenase
LFT	liver function test
LH	luteinising hormone
LHRH	luteinising hormone releasing hormone
LIF	left iliac fossa
LRTI	lower respiratory tract infection
LMWH	low molecular weight heparin
LUQ	left upper quandrant
MCP	metacarpophalangeal joint
MCV	mean corpuscular volume
MDT	multidisciplinary team
MI	myocardial infarction
MRI	magnetic resonance imaging
MSU	mid-stream urine
NBM	nil by mouth
NG	nasogastric
NO	nitrous oxide
NSAIDs	non-steroidal anti-inflammatory drugs
OGD	oesophagogastroduodenoscopy
OM	osteomyelitis
OSA	obstructive sleep apnoea
PA	postero anterior
PDA	patent ductus arteriosus
PE	pulmonary embolism

PET	positron emission tomography
PIP	proximal interphalangeal joint
PPI	proton pump inhibitor
PR	per rectum
PTH	parathyroid hormone
PVD	peripheral vascular disease
RIF	right iliac fossa
RR	respiratory rate
RTA	road traffic accident
RTC	road traffic collision
RUQ	right upper quandrant
SAH	subarachnoid haemorrhage
SLE	systemic lupus erythematosis
SOL	space occupying lesion
STI	sexually transmitted infection
TB	tuberculosis
TMJ	temperomandibular joint
TNM	tumour, node, metastasis
TRUS	transrectal ultrasound
TSH	thyroid stimulating hormone
TURP	transurethral resection of prostate
U+E	urea and electolytes
URTI	upper respiratory tract infection
USS	ultrasound scan
UTI	urinary tract infection
VSD	ventriculoseptal defect
VTE	venous thromboembolism

Chapter 1

General surgery

Scott Castell

SAQs

1 A 22-year-old girl comes to see you in the GP surgery. She complains of a month-long history of worsening tremor, palpitations and swelling in the midline of her neck.

   a Give three possible causes of a lump in the midline of the neck. (3 marks)

   b Through history and examination, how would you determine the cause of the lump? Give four factors in the history and four in the examination. (4 marks)

   c You ascertain the lump is most likely thyroid in origin. Name two different types of thyroid lump. (2 marks)

   d Give three ways you would further investigate the thyroid lump. (3 marks)

   e Not all thyroid lumps require surgery. Give two indications for surgical removal of the thyroid. (2 marks)

   f Why is hoarseness of the voice a complication of thyroid surgery? (1 mark)

2 A 57-year-old lady presents to her GP with a 2-week history of vague abdominal discomfort and back pain. Her past medical history includes a fractured wrist 2 weeks previously. She comes in with her husband who comments that she has been 'acting strange' lately.

   a Routine blood tests show that her serum calcium level is 3.0 mmol/L. Give three other symptoms you should ask about. (2 marks)

   b You admit her to hospital, what four other investigations would you request? (4 marks)

   c Results show that she has primary hyperparathyroidism. What three blood results could you expect? (3 marks)

   d What is the commonest cause of primary hyperparathyroidism? (1 mark)

   e It is decided that surgical management of this lady is appropriate. What three complications may arise from surgery? (3 marks)

3 A 46-year-old man presents to A&E after recently being discharged following an explorative laparoscopy. He complains his scar is not healing. Examination reveals a swollen, erythematous area around one of his laparoscopy wounds.

    a Name four signs associated with any inflammatory response. (4 marks)

    b You diagnose the lump as a post-surgical cutaneous abscess. Give three ways in which you would further investigate this. (3 marks)

    c What is the definitive curative treatment for cutaneous abscesses? (1 mark)

    d Name three risk factors for forming an abscess. (3 marks)

    e Name three complications of abscess formation. (3 marks)

4 A 30-year-old gentleman presents to A&E after injuring his finger. He works on a construction site and says that he caught his finger in a drill. Examination reveals an open wound at the tip of his left middle finger that will require cleaning and suturing.

    a Give three methods you may use to control the pain for the patient to facilitate cleaning and suturing. (3 marks)

    b Explain the mechanism of action for local anaesthetic (LA) agents. (3 marks)

    c What other agent would you normally administer along with LA, but is contraindicated in this case, and why is it contraindicated? (2 marks)

    d Name three types of LA agent. (3 marks)

    e When the LA agent is administered, the skin of the finger becomes warm and dry – what is the explanation for this? (2 marks)

    f What are the benefits of administering local anaesthesia over general anaesthesia? (4 marks)

5 Frank is a 65-year-old man who has severe osteoarthritis. He requires a hip replacement under general anaesthetic (GA).

    a Explain the triad of general anaesthesia. (3 marks)

    b What are the three phases of general anaesthesia? (3 marks)

    c Induction of anaesthesia can be either IV or inhalation. Which is most common, and what induction agents are widely used? (4 marks)

    d What physiological markers are used for monitoring during a GA? (4 marks)

    e As the muscle relaxant is administered in to Frank, he appears to shake and his muscles contract. He then relaxes. This is common during induction. What is happening? (3 marks)

   f   Give three potential complications of general
anaesthesia. (3 marks)

6 Margaret is a 62-year-old lady who is due to have a routine laparoscopic
cholecystectomy. She meets the anaesthetist before the operation, who
performs a full pre-operative assessment.

   a   List four main aims of the pre-operative assessment. (4 marks)

   b   Margaret had a myocardial infarction (MI) 4 years
previously, and is known to suffer from mild ischaemic
heart disease (IHD). What four pre-operative
investigations would you consider for her? (4 marks)

   c   ASA Classification is a scale determined by the
American Society of Anesthesiologists. It describes a
patient's risk for anaesthetic. Briefly describe the levels
within this classification. (5 marks)

   d   Assessment of a patient's airway is an important aspect
of pre-operative assessment. Give three factors that
contribute to a potentially difficult intubation. (3 marks)

   e   What is the name given to the scoring system for
determining difficult intubation? (1 mark)

7 Ben is a 24-year-old man who comes in for a diagnostic laparoscopy. The
surgeon meets with him prior to the operation to obtain consent.

   a   Explain the term 'informed consent'. (2 marks)

   b   In order to give consent, Ben must be determined to
have capacity. Give four aspects of capacity. (4 marks)

   c   List two circumstances in which someone else can give
consent on behalf of the patient. (2 marks)

   d   During the operation, the surgeon decides that he will
have to convert to an open procedure. He performs
a laparotomy. Under what circumstances is this
considered legal? (2 marks)

8 A 32-year-old man presents to A&E after falling off a ladder at work.
He landed on a 100 mm nail sticking out of a plank of wood. The nail is
embedded in the anterior abdominal wall. After stabilisation in A&E, you
are part of the surgical team asked to review the patient.

   a   Give four aspects of your initial assessment of this patient. (4 marks)

   b   Examination reveals that the patient has peritonitis and
is shocked. What is the likely cause? (1 mark)

   c   Give four investigations you would consider. (4 marks)

   d   What would you expect to see on an erect chest X-ray? (1 mark)

   e   What would be the surgical procedure of choice for this
patient? (1 mark)

9 Joanne is a 45-year-old lady who attends A&E complaining of stomach pain following a car accident yesterday. History reveals that her car slid on ice and she hit a lamppost at approximately 20 mph. She thinks she hit her stomach on the steering wheel, and complains of pain in her left upper quadrant (LUQ).

  a Give three organs at risk in this area.   (3 marks)
  b Further examination reveals severe tenderness in the
     LUQ and also pain in her left shoulder. Explain the
     shoulder tip pain.   (2 marks)
  c Give two normal functions of the spleen.   (2 marks)
  d What is the likely cause for splenic injury in this case?   (1 mark)
  e Give four causes of splenomegaly.   (4 marks)
  f Joanne becomes hypotensive and tachycardic, and the
     decision is made to operate. She requires a splenectomy.
     Give four aspects of post-operative advice that should be
     given to the patient.   (4 marks)

10 David is a 15-year-old boy who presents to A&E with vague abdominal pain, which is now moving to his right side and he is reported by his mother to be off his food. Examination reveals he is tachycardic and dehydrated. He looks in obvious discomfort and has pain in his right iliac fossa (RIF).

  a Give the two most likely differential diagnoses.   (2 marks)
  b You examine David. What is Rovsing's Sign?   (1 mark)
  c Give four aspects of your initial management.   (4 marks)
  d What is the definitive treatment of choice?   (1 mark)
  e Give three potential complications of acute appendicitis.   (3 marks)

EMQs

  A Bupivicaine
  B Adrenaline
  C Brachial plexus block
  D Lidocaine
  E Procaine

  1 Has a short onset of action and is most commonly used in A&E.
  2 Has a short duration of action and is used commonly for minor surgical
         procedures.
  3 Is used in epidural anaesthesia.
  4 Will cause temporary paraesthesia of the hand and arm.
  5 Causes vasoconstriction and prevents spread around the body.

A Rovsing's Sign
B Umbilical pain
C Ectopic pregnancy
D Mesenteric adenitis
E Perforation

6 Initial onset of pain caused by irritation of visceral nerve fibres.
7 A differential diagnosis in a young woman.
8 A shocked patient with guarding and rebound tenderness.
9 Pain in the RIF when the left iliac fossa (LIF) is pressed.
10 Abdominal pain in a child 2 weeks following coryzal symptoms.

A Congestive heart failure
B A patient with mild systemic disease
C Patient refusal with informed consent
D Gastrectomy
E Cholecystectomy

11 Will require a group and save prior to surgery.
12 Is a contraindication to surgery.
13 Signifies ASA Grade II.
14 Will require a cross-match prior to surgery.
15 Is a significant comorbidity in all surgical patients.

A Incision and drainage
B Pilonidal abscess
C Antibiotics
D Empyema
E Perianal abscess

16 Is defined as a collection within a pre-existing cavity.
17 May be a complication of Crohn's disease.
18 Occurs in the natal cleft.
19 Is the treatment of choice for an abscess.
20 Should be used in cases where surrounding cellulitis is evident.

A Capacity must be ascertained before consent
B Can give informed consent
C Life-saving surgery deemed appropriate
D Surgery is not appropriate
E Prior consent must be obtained

21 A life-threatening burst abdominal aortic aneurysm (AAA), in an unconscious 50-year-old male.
22 A patient who is under 16 and understands the procedure.
23 A 22-year-old patient refusing non-life threatening surgery.
24 A patient who is over 18 but suffers from a learning disability.
25 A major change in plan during the procedure, which is not life-threatening.

MCQs

1 What is the commonest cause of hyperthyroidism?
    a   Hashimoto's thyroiditis
    b   Congenital thyroid abnormalities
    c   Graves' disease
    d   Surgical resection of thyroid
    e   Infection

2 What is the action of suxamethonium?
    a   Analgesic
    b   Acetylcholinesterase inhibitor
    c   Paralytic agent
    d   Acetylcholine stimulator
    e   Alpha-blocker

3 What is the key indication for laparotomy in patients suffering penetrating abdominal trauma?
    a   Shock
    b   Peritonitis
    c   Low O_2 sats
    d   Vomiting
    e   Metabolic acidosis

4 On abdominal examination, where would you expect to find an enlarged spleen?
    a   Right upper quadrant (RUQ)
    b   LUQ extending to the LIF
    c   LUQ extending to RUQ
    d   RUQ extending to RIF
    e   LUQ extending to RIF

5   What is the anatomical location of the parathyroid glands?
   a   Inferior to the thyroid gland
   b   Posterior to the thyroid gland
   c   Superior to the thyroid gland
   d   Inferior to the hyoid bone
   e   Lateral to the thyroid gland

6   Which of the features below are indicative of small bowel on abdominal X-ray?
   a   Haustrations
   b   Appendices epiploicae
   c   Taenia coli
   d   'Coffee bean' sign
   e   Valvulae conniventes

7   What is the most effective treatment for acute appendicitis?
   a   Aggressive fluid replacement
   b   Antibiotics
   c   Analgesia
   d   Surgical removal
   e   Watch and wait

8   What is the first-line antibiotic of choice in a skin abscess?
   a   Erythromycin
   b   Flucloxacillin
   c   Co-Amoxiclav
   d   Teiocoplanin
   e   None, incision and drainage should be performed

9   What is the age at which a patient can legally refuse treatment?
   a   16
   b   18
   c   20
   d   12
   e   21

10 What is rapid sequence induction?
   a   Anaesthetising a patient whilst preparing an operation site
   b   A term used to anaesthetise a patient who has not been starved and is at risk of aspiration
   c   Using volatile induction instead of IV
   d   Intubating with a laryngeal mask airway
   e   Insertion of a tracheostomy

Answers

SAQs

1 a Dermoid cyst
Thyroid mass
Branchial cyst
Pharngyeal pouch
Thyroglossal cyst

    b History – onset, duration, pain, colour change, size (fluctuation), associated symptoms, systemic symptoms
Examination – location, size, shape, consistency, movement on swallowing, movement on protrusion of tongue, lymphadenopathy, retrosternal percussion for retrosternal expansion of the thyroid, auscultation to listen for carotid bruit, if carotid body tumour

    c Single nodular goitre
Toxic multinodular goitre
Smooth non-toxic goitre
Malignant thyroid tumour

    d Bloods – full blood count (FBC), urea and electrolytes (U+E), thyroid function test (TFT) (tri-iodothyronine (T3), thyroxine (T4), thyroid stimulating hormone (TSH))
Ultrasound – to assess whether it is a solid lump, cystic, or follicular.
Radioisotope scans – shows areas of hotspots/coldspots, depending on over/under functioning thyroid tissue
Fine needle aspiration

    e Compression symptoms – airway compromise, dysphagia, pain
Cosmetic reasons
Uncontrolled hyperthyroidism
Malignancy

    f The recurrent laryngeal nerves supply motor innervation to the glottic folds, which lie posterolateral to the lobes of the thyroid. During surgery these nerves can be injured. If this happens to one of these nerves the vocal fold becomes paralysed in a semi-abducted position. When air flows through the folds during phonation, it becomes turbulent causing a hoarse voice.

Neck swelling is a presentation with many different causes. It is important to take a full history and perform a thorough examination to rule out or confirm potentially serious conditions. A thyroid swelling may not always present with a thyrotoxic patient. Thyroid cancer can be aggressive and has many forms, including papillary, follicular, anaplastic, medullary, and lymphoma. Many of these forms will require adjuvant chemotherapy alongside surgical resection.

2 a Bone pain or fractures
      Renal stones
      Abdominal pains
      Psychiatric symptoms
   b FBC, LFT, serum PTH levels, albumin, U+E, phosphate
      24 hour urinary calcium
      Spinal X-ray
      Kidneys, ureter, bladder (KUB) X-ray
      ECG
   c Raised parathyroid hormone (PTH)
      Raised serum calcium
      Low phosphate
   d Parathyroid adenoma (85% of cases)
   e Infection
      Recurrent laryngeal nerve palsy
      Expanding haematoma causing tracheal compression
      Hypocalcaemia
      Hypoparathyroidism

Primary hyperparathyroidism is often an incidental finding without symptomatic hypercalcaemia. The commonest cause is a single adenoma in the parathyroid gland, in 85% of cases. The remaining 15% are caused by multiple adenomas, and rarely parathyroid carcinoma. Hypercalcaemia results when overproduction of PTH occurs. PTH acts to reabsorb calcium from bone, and from the kidney which lead to the symptoms mentioned above. Hypercalaemia can also present with very vague, non-specific symptoms which are easy to miss, or attribute to another condition.

3 a Rubor – redness
      Dolor – pain
      Calor – warmth
      Tumour – swelling
      Function laesa – loss of function
   b History and examination
      Bloods – FBC, U+E, C-reactive protease (CRP)
      Swab – for culture
   c Incision and drainage
   d Bacterial contamination of surgical site
      Diabetes
      Previous abscess formation
      Immunosuppression
      Alcoholism
      Chemotherapy

    e Chronic abscess formation
       Sinus formation
       Cellulitus
       Fistula formation
       Bacteraemia and sepsis

An abscess is a collection of pus and both live and dead neutrophils, macrophages and bacteria. It may also include dead tissue. Cutaneous skin abscesses are usually rare following surgery but can occur spontaneously in obese, diabetic or immunosuppressed patients. The commonest bacterial contamination is with *Staphylococcus aureus* as it is normally present on skin, but antibiotics are not routinely given unless cellulitis is also present. Incision and drainage is curative. Inadequate drainage may lead to the build-up of granulation tissue and chronic abscess formation.

4 a Entonox
       Opioid analgesics
       LA – digital nerve block
    b Binds to Na+ and K+ channels on nerve cell membrane
       Prevents depolarisation of cell by outflux of Na+ ions
       This prevents propagation of action potential by inhibiting depolarisation of neighbouring cells
    c Adrenaline to combat the vasodilator effect of the anaesthetic and prevent excessive bleeding
       Contraindicated in terminal digits or the penis due to inhibition of single route of blood flow, causing ischaemia in the digit
    d Procaine
       Lidocaine
       Bupivicaine
       Marcaine
       Cocaine
       Prilocaine
       Novocaine
       Levobupivicaine
    e The LA agent not only blocks somatic pain fibres but also autonomic nerve fibres, thus inhibiting a sympathetic response leading to a lack of sweating and peripheral vasodilation.
    f Lower anaesthetic risk – i.e. in patients with multiple co-morbidities
       Shorter hospital stay
       Lower risk of adverse effects
       Can be administered by emergency doctors, not only anaesthetists
       Fewer contraindications

LA provides a reliable alternative to general anaesthesia in providing pre-operative analgesia in both minor and major surgery. It can be administered via infiltration into the surrounding tissue, i.e. when suturing a wound or it can be administered into the surrounding nerve plexus. This is called a nerve block and is very useful to anaesthetise specific areas of the body. Common blocks include digital nerve blocks, caudal blocks and brachial plexus blocks. Regional anaesthesia is another form of local anaesthesia and includes common procedures such as an epidural, and spinal blocks. The most commonly used LA agent is lidocaine and it differs only from others in terms of duration of action. Heavy bupivacaine is used in epidural and spinal blocks to aid infiltration of anaesthetic agent towards the legs and away from the diaphragm.

5 a The three imperative factors which allow for successful anaesthetic are:
paralysis – to prevent movement which would inhibit surgery
unconsciousness – to enable the patient to not remember the surgical event
analgesia – so the patient does not feel any pain, which would be intolerable without the anaesthetic

  b Induction
Maintenance
Recovery

  c IV
Propofol
Thiopental
Etomidate
Ketamine

  d Heart rate
Blood pressure
End-tidal CO_2
Mean alveolar concentration
Oxygen saturations
Positive end-expiratory pressure

  e The muscle relaxant administered is a depolarising muscle relaxant that works by depolarising all the nerve cells, and then blocking them. The muscles contract as they are depolarised and then become still. A type of depolarising muscle relaxant is Suxamethonium.

  f Post-operative nausea and vomiting
Inadequate analgesia
Respiratory depression
Allergic reaction
Malignant hyperthermia
Retained consciousness

General anaesthesia is described as a process rather than an event, and hence has very important steps that require close monitoring. Alongside the critical triad of anaesthesia, other medications are given to enable a smooth anaesthetic process, these include antiemetics, anxiolytics and antisialogues to reduce secretions and decrease airway obstruction. The patient is induced, normally using an IV induction agent, and the airway is then managed via endotracheal tube, or laryngeal mask airway. The anaesthetic is maintained by volatile inhalation agent, whilst analgesia is maintained by opioid analgesics. Recovery involves stopping the anaesthetic agent, and occasionally reversing the muscle relaxant.

6 a   Build relationship with patient
Determine fitness for anaesthetic
Discuss options (LA vs. GA)
Plan to hold or stop patient's current medications
Post-operative analgesia
Determine any previous problems with anaesthetic – post-operative nausea and vomiting, intolerance

b   Full history and physical examination
Blood pressure
Blood tests – FBC, renal function, cholesterol, glucose, LFT
ECG
Chest X-ray
Echo
Exercise stress test

c   I – a fit patient with no co-morbidities
II – a patient with mild systemic disease
III – a patient with severe systemic disease limiting activity
IV – a patient with a severe systemic disease that is incapacitating and a constant threat to life
V – a moribound patient not expected to survive more than 24 hours

d   Short neck
Previous intubation difficulties
Obesity
Rheumatoid arthritis
C-spine trauma
Limited neck movement
Prominent upper incisors
Micrognathia
Congenital deformities – Pierre Robin, Treacher-Collins
Facial trauma

e   Mallampati Classification

Pre-operative assessment is an important part of the anaesthetic process. The aim is to air any concerns that both the patient and the anaesthetist have. The patient must be made aware of what is going to happen. Their analgesia requirement must be taken into consideration, as standard analgesia cannot be applied to all patients. The anaesthetist must take a full medical and surgical history to elicit any potential problems that may occur during induction, maintenance or recovery from anaesthesia.

Respiratory conditions, cardiovascular conditions, and hepato-renal conditions are particularly important to discuss.

Pre-operative investigations will help quantify disease and allow for the anaesthetist to plan more precisely.

7 a An agreement to a procedure or treatment given with prior knowledge and understanding of risks and benefits of said procedure.

b Ability to take in information given
Ability to retain the information
Ability to weigh up the information and make a decision
Ability to communicate this decision

c If the patient is determined not to have capacity then it can be decided by the surgeon
If the patient is considered a 'minor' (less than 16-years-old) and does not understand the procedure

d If the surgeon had already obtained consent for the laparotomy prior to the operation or it is deemed a life-saving procedure. It is common to include this as a potential risk for the surgery, to allow the surgeon scope for performing the surgery successfully.

Informed consent is a complex subject. It is important to give the patient information concerning all the potential risks and benefits of the procedure. It is equally as important to make sure that the patient understands what you are saying, and has adequate, pressure-free time to come to their own decision. If you are unclear as to whether a person can consent for their procedure, it is best to contact your senior doctor.

8 a **A**irway, **B**reathing, **C**irculation, **D**isability, **E**xposure
History – force of trauma, what exactly happened, what has happened up until now, any significant past medical history
Examination – examine site of stab wound, is there peritonitis (guarding, rigidity, rebound tenderness), do per rectum (PR) exam – blood on finger
Observations – blood pressure, pulse, respiratory rate, saturations

b Perforation of bowel

    c   Bloods – FBC, U+E, LFT, clotting, cross-match four units, amylase
          Erect chest X-ray, abdominal X-ray
          Abdominal CT
          Rigid sigmoidoscopy
    d   Air under the diaphragm indicative of bowel perforation
    e   Emergency laparotomy.

Abdominal stab wounds have to be managed concurrently with history taking, especially if there are signs of shock and the patient is obviously unstable. They will be managed according to acute trauma life support (ATLS) guidelines initially by the emergency team. Examination is important in deciding if internal organ injury is present. Laparotomy is indicated in all incidences of abdominal trauma where peritonitis is present. Other indications include gunshot wounds, continuing shock despite resuscitation, multi-patterned bruising, and sub-phrenic gas on erect chest X-ray.

9   a   Spleen
          Pancreas
          Stomach
          Large bowel
          Lung
    b   Inflammation of an organ in the LUQ can lead to diaphragmatic irritation, and since the visceral nerve supply to the diaphragm is the same as the cutaneous nerve supply of the shoulder, a sensation known as referred pain can occur.
    c   Filtration of red blood cells
          Breakdown red blood cells
          Store monocytes
          Storage and release of lymphocytes in humoral or cell-mediated immunity
          Blood reservoir
          Eradication of encapsulated organisms
    d   Rib fracture
    e   Epstein Barr virus (EBV)
          Hepatitis
          Leptospirosis
          AIDS
          Malignancy
          Lymphoma
          Systemic lupus erythematosis (SLE)
          Rheumatoid arthritis
          Leukaemia

f   She will have to have immunisations against haemophilus, meningoccocal and pneumococcal bacteria as these are encapsulated bacteria, which cannot be broken down without a spleen.
Warn her of the dangers of overwhelming post-splenectomy infection and sepsis.
She will need lifelong prophylactic antibiotics, and should seek hospital advice if she develops an infection despite these measures.
She should be counselled about the risks of overseas travel – malaria, and animal bites.
She should carry a card or pendant to warn health professionals of her asplenia.

Splenic injury is almost always caused by blunt trauma, especially deceleration injuries, and is normally protected by the rib cage in the LUQ. It can also occur iatrogenically from colonoscopy, or spontaneous rupture can occur in infective mononucleosis.

Shoulder tip pain is classical of splenic injury or enlargement, as it irritates the overlying diaphragm.

Upon assessing a patient, you should be looking for signs of splenic rupture such as hypotension and tachycardia. They may also have signs of peritonism. In these patients, it is usually contraindicated to investigate with CT and they should be taken straight to theatre.

It is important that patients are aware of the complications of a splenectomy and should be counselled correctly on vaccinations, antibiotic prophylaxis and foreign travel.

10 a   Appendicitis
Mesenteric adenitis
b   Pain worse in the RIF when the LIF is palpated
c   Take blood – FBC, U+E, CRP, LFT
Urine M, C+S
Make the patient nil by mouth (NBM)
Start IV fluids
Abdominal X-ray and erect chest X-ray to rule out perforation
Analgesia
d   Laparoscopic or open appendicectomy
e   Appendix mass
Appendix abscess
Sepsis
Persistent ileus
Perforation
Peritonitis

Acute appendicitis is the commonest surgical emergency. Classical presentation is with initial peri-umbilical pain that then localises to the RIF. This is because initial appendix inflammation stimulates the surrounding visceral peritoneum (which has the common nerve root T10 which also innervates the dermatome surrounding the umbilicus). As further inflammation develops, there is stimulation of the parietal peritoneum causing more localised pain.

EMQs

1	**D**	10	**D**	19	**A**
2	**E**	11	**E**	20	**C**
3	**A**	12	**C**	21	**C**
4	**C**	13	**B**	22	**B**
5	**B**	14	**D**	23	**D**
6	**B**	15	**A**	24	**A**
7	**C**	16	**D**	25	**E**
8	**E**	17	**E**		
9	**A**	18	**B**		

MCQs

1 c – Hyperthyroidism is most commonly caused by Graves' disease, however it may also be due to a toxic thyroid adenoma, toxic multinodular goitre, thyroiditis, or a pituitary adenoma.

2 c – Suxamethonium is a paralytic-induction agent which inhibits the action of acetylcholine at the neuromuscular junction.

3 a and b – Any patient with penetrating abdominal trauma may have internal organ damage. If a patient is peritonitic and in shock then exploratory laparotomy is indicated as a first-line investigation. Only a stable patient may be scanned.

4 e – The spleen is 3 cm by 5 cm by 7 cm and lies under the left 9th and 11th ribs. When enlarged, it spreads to the RIF.

5 b – The four parathyroid glands typically lie posterior to the thyroid gland, however, they can descend into the mediastinum.

6 e – Small bowel is identified by being central, with the presence of valvulae conniventes.

7 d – Appendicitis requires prompt surgical excision.

8 e – An abscess should be drained aseptically in theatre, with thorough wash-out. Antibiotics are not indicated unless there is marked cellulitis or necrotising fasciitis.

9 a – Patients may consent for treatment at any age, if Gillick and Fraser competent, however, they cannot refuse treatment until the age of 16.
10 b – Rapid sequence induction is done to prevent aspiration, by applying cricoid pressure during intubation.

Chapter 2

Lower GI surgery

Pandora Spillman-Henham

SAQs

1 A 28-year-old lady is seen in clinic regarding pain on defaecation. You diagnose an anal fissure.

    a Give two symptoms she may describe in her history.   (2 marks)

    b What position in the anus are anal fissures most likely to occur?   (1 mark)

    c Name a situation where one may form in the anterior wall.   (1 mark)

    d Anal fissures are usually shallow and heal without intervention. Deeper ones are more problematic and do not heal as easily. Explain the pathology which leads to this.   (2 marks)

    e Anal fissures can be managed medically or surgically depending on their severity. Name two medical treatments.   (2 marks)

    f Anal dilation has previously been used as a surgical management option. Explain why this is no longer performed.   (1 mark)

    g What is the current choice of surgical intervention for anal fissures?   (1 mark)

2 A 70-year-old lady presents with colicky abdominal pain and bloody stools.

    a Give two aspects of this patient's history you would like to illicit.   (2 marks)

    b What investigation is most useful in diagnosing a colorectal carcinoma and why?   (2 marks)

    c Colorectal carcinoma is classified according to the modified Dukes classification, Dukes A to D. Define these four grades.   (4 marks)

    d Name two predisposing factors for colorectal cancer.   (2 marks)

    e There are a number of surgical options depending on the location of the malignancy. State the likely locations of malignancy which the following operations would be

used for: (4 marks)
- ➤ right hemicolectomy
- ➤ left hemicolectomy
- ➤ abdomino-perineal resection
- ➤ anterior resection.

3 A 23-year-old female presents to the surgical unit. She is complaining of diarrhoea and abdominal pain. On further questioning, she tells you that she has noticed some blood in her stools.

    a Give three differential diagnoses other than Crohn's disease. (3 marks)

    b What two investigations would you request if you suspected this may be Crohn's disease? (2 marks)

    c Which part of the gastrointestinal (GI) tract does Crohn's disease affect, and where is the most common area? (1 mark)

    d Fistulas are a complication of Crohn's disease. Describe two common types of fistula associated with Crohn's disease. (2 marks)

    e There are a number of extra-intestinal complications associated with inflammatory bowel disease. Name two of them. (2 marks)

    f Name two medications commonly used in the management of Crohn's disease. (2 marks)

    g Give one reason why a patient may undergo surgery for Crohn's disease. (1 mark)

4 A 54-year-old woman is seen by her GP with a lump in her groin.

    a Give two differential diagnoses other than a hernia. (2 marks)

    b The lump is currently painless and reducible although she sometimes experiences a pulling sensation at the site. You think this may be a femoral hernia. Where would you expect to find a femoral hernia? (2 marks)

    c Anatomically what forms the four borders of the femoral canal? (4 marks)

    d The same lady presents to the surgical unit 2 weeks later. The lump is now irreducible. What may have happened to her hernia? (1 mark)

    e What three accompanying features would you expect with your diagnosis? (3 marks)

    f Explain the management for this acute emergency. (1 mark)

5 A 64-year-old gentleman visits his GP with rectal bleeding. He says that the blood is fresh. There has been some on the toilet paper and some in the pan.

    a Other than haemorrhoids give three differential diagnoses for his symptoms. (3 marks)

    b What three further questions would you like to ask? (3 marks)

    c Name two risks factors for haemorrhoids. (2 marks)

    d Define the four grades of haemorrhoids. (4 marks)

    e Haemorrhoids can be treated medically or surgically. Give three interventions to manage haemorrhoids. (3 marks)

6 A 28-year-old female presents to A&E with abdominal pain. She reports diarrhoea with 4–6 bowel movements per day. She is passing both blood and mucus with her stool. Her Hb is 9.8, MCV is normal. Her WCC is 13.5 and CRP is 104. She reports a long history of these symptoms, on and off for years.

    a What is the most likely diagnosis? (1 mark)

    b Patients with inflammatory bowel disease may have signs unrelated to the GI tract (GIT). Name three of these signs. (3 marks)

    c Ulcerative colitis only affects the colon and rectum. It does not affect the bowel proximal to the ileo-caecal valve. What is it called when only the rectum is involved? (1 mark)

    d Define pancolitis. (1 mark)

    e What is found on rectal biopsy in a patient with ulcerative colitis? (1 mark)

    f The medications used in the management of ulcerative colitis are the same as in Crohn's disease. Surgery can also be performed. Why is surgery for ulcerative colitis more successful than in Crohn's disease? (1 mark)

7 A 26-year-old female attends the GP saying that she can feel a small lump at her anus. You examine her and see a lump which is a small flap of skin. You diagnose a skin tag.

    a What are anal skin tags? (1 mark)

    b Give two causes for anal skin tags. (2 marks)

    c What is a sentinel skin tag? (1 mark)

    d Name two pathologies associated with skin tags. (2 marks)

    e What are the symptoms associated with skin tags? (1 mark)

    f Skin tags usually do not require treatment although they may point to an underlying pathology. Give two interventions which can be used if a skin tag becomes large or troublesome. (2 marks)

    g In what situation would you like to biopsy these lesions? (1 mark)

8 A 29-year-old man is admitted to the surgical admissions unit. He is complaining of pain around the anus. He says that the pain becomes worse on defecation and that he can feel a lump which is painful. He has a temperature of 37.9°. You suspect from this history that he has a perianal abscess.

    a Give three signs or symptoms you expect to find on examination. (3 marks)

    b Where does the infection originate? (1 mark)

    c Name two common organisms implicated in abscess formation. (2 marks)

    d List two diseases which are associated with perianal abscesses. (2 marks)

    e What is the best management option for an abscess? (1 mark)

    f Explain why an abscess should be left open. (1 mark)

9 A 54-year-old man visits his GP. He has noticed a lump under a scar from abdominal surgery he had a few years previously. The lump is soft and painless.

    a What is the most likely diagnosis? (1 mark)

    b Give a definition for this diagnosis. (1 mark)

    c There are a number of risk factors for this. Name three. (3 marks)

    d What is the potential complication of this condition? Explain why it is less likely to happen in this type of pathology. (2 marks)

    e Name two available management options. (2 marks)

10 A 78-year-old female is admitted to the surgical admission unit with fresh PR bleeding which has been intermittent for a few days. She is also complaining of abdominal pain in her left lower abdomen.

    a Give two differential diagnoses. (2 marks)

    b Give two further questions you would ask to focus your diagnosis. (2 marks)

    c On examination, she has a temperature of 38°. Her white cell count is 18. She is very tender in her LIF. On PR there is an empty rectum and the glove is clean. What is the most likely diagnosis? (1 mark)

    d Explain the pathology behind this diagnosis. (2 marks)

    e What non-invasive imaging test would you like to request for this patient? (1 mark)

    f Give three aspects of this patient's management you would initiate. (3 marks)

    g Despite your treatment, you notice that her white cell count is now 20 and her temperature has been spiking. What is this likely to be a sign of? (1 mark)

11 A 65-year-old lady presents to her GP with recurrent urinary tract infections (UTIs). She has had repeated courses of antibiotics but the infection keeps returning. She says that recently she has noticed some brown material in her urine. You suspect a colovesical fistula.

a	Define a fistula.	(1 mark)
b	Define a colovesical fistula.	(1 mark)
c	Where does the fistula usually occur?	(1 mark)
d	Name two other common types of GI fistula.	(2 marks)
e	Name two specific pathologies associated with colovesical fistulae.	(2 marks)
f	Give two investigations that may be performed to diagnose this condition.	(2 marks)
g	What is the treatment option for this condition?	(1 mark)

12 A 65-year-old gentlemen presents to A&E with a lump in his groin. This lump is soft and painless. On examination, it is located above and medial to the pubic tubercle and the lump is reducible. You decide that this is likely to be an inguinal hernia.

a	Name the structures which form the roof and floor of the inguinal canal.	(2 marks)
b	What two structures pass through this inguinal canal in a woman?	(2 marks)
c	Name the three fascial layers of the spermatic cord and where they are derived from.	(3 marks)
d	From where do direct hernias enter the inguinal canal?	(1 mark)
e	From where do indirect hernias enter the inguinal canal?	(1 mark)
f	How is it possible to illicit the difference between a direct and indirect inguinal hernia?	(1 mark)
g	Which type of inguinal hernia is more prone to strangulation?	(1 mark)

EMQs

Match the most likely diagnosis with the presentation below:
A Diverticulitis
B Anal fissure
C Anal fistula
D Anal skin tag
E Bowel malignancy
F Haemorrhoids
G Crohn's disease
H Ulcerative colitis
I Angiodysplasia

1   A 70-year-old lady is admitted with fresh blood PR, mixed with her stool. She has lost 1 stone in weight over the last 6 months. She has not had any abdominal pain and there is no pain on defecation.
2   A 43-year-old man is admitted with rectal pain. He suffers from constipation and tells you that he has had fresh PR bleeding mostly on the toilet paper and a little in the pan. PR examination is very painful and you notice what looks like a sentinel skin tag.
3   An 83-year-old lady is admitted with PR bleeding. The blood is fresh but of a minimal amount. On examination, her temperature is 38.2° and she is very tender in her LIF.
4   A 35-year-old smoker is admitted with PR bleeding and abdominal pain. She has been experiencing diarrhoea, and passing mucus with her bowel movements. She has had a colonoscopy which shows pathology in a number of parts of her bowel.
5   A 26-year-old man reports fresh PR bleeding which is not mixed with his stool. He says that defecation is painful. On examination, you notice a number of lumps around his anus which are at the 3, 7 and 11 o'clock positions.

Match the diagnosis with the history below:
A   Femoral hernia
B   Indirect inguinal hernia
C   Direct inguinal hernia
D   Spigelian hernia
E   Gluteal hernia
F   Paraumbilical hernia
G   Umbilical hernia
H   Incisional hernia
I   Epigastric hernia

6   A 30-year-old female with an irreducible lump lateral to the pubic tubercle.
7   A 62-year-old man with a history of a right hemicolectomy, with a large swelling through the scar site.
8   A 2-year-old boy with a persistent swelling around the navel since birth.
9   A 43-year-old man with a reducible hernia, which is maintained with direct pressure on the internal ring.
10 A protrusion through the right side of the abdomen lateral to the rectus sheath.

Please match the most appropriate procedure with the patient description:
A Subtotal colectomy
B Panproctocolectomy
C Right hemicolectomy
D Left hemicolectomy
E Anterior resection
F Abdomino-perineal resection
G Hartmann's procedure
H Sigmoid colectomy

11 A patient with ulcerative colitis not resolving with medical treatment.
12 A 70-year-old woman admitted with peritonitis secondary to perforated sigmoid diverticular disease.
13 A patient with localised rectal cancer.
14 A 60-year-old man with a tumour found in the descending colon on bowel screening.
15 An otherwise healthy 60-year-old lady with chronic diverticular disease.
16 A patient with a tumour in the ascending colon.

Match the description below with the staging for colorectal cancer:
A Dukes A
B Dukes B
C Dukes C
D Dukes D

17 A tumour with lymph node involvement.
18 A tumour confined to the bowel wall.
19 A tumour which has spread to the liver.
20 A tumour spreading through the wall of the bowel.

Please match the structure with the description:
A Inguinal ligament
B Conjoint tendon
C Scarpa's fascia
D Ilioinguinal nerve
E Camper's fascia
F Testicular artery
G Lacunar ligament

21 The second layer of fascia on the anterior abdominal wall.
22 Contained within the spermatic cord.
23 Superior border of the femoral triangle.
24 Formed from the transversus abdominus and internal oblique.
25 Medial border of the femoral canal.

MCQs

1 What two things from the list below would you expect to find on examination in a patient suffering with an anal fissure?
a   Sentinel pile
b   Erythematous area around the anus
c   Painful PR examination
d   Multiple skin tags around the anus
e   Abscess

2 Which of the following is a characteristic of Crohn's disease?
a   Affects only the large bowel
b   Bowel wall becomes thickened and produces a 'cobblestone effect'
c   Inflammation affects the mucosa only
d   It is associated with non-smokers
e   Bowel wall becomes thin

3 Colovesical fistulae are more common in women, with a ratio of:
a   2:1
b   3:1
c   4:1
d   5:1
e   6:1

4 Which of the following is NOT an extra-intestinal sign of inflammatory bowel disease?
a   Clubbing
b   Pyoderma gangrenosum
c   Episcleritis
d   Spider naevi
e   Ankylosing spondylitis

5 Strangulation is not common in which of the following hernias?
a   Femoral hernia
b   Incisional hernia
c   Inguinal hernia
d   Paraumbilical hernia
e   Spigelian hernia

6 Which is not a common characteristic of haemorrhoids?
  a PR bleeding
  b Rectal pain
  c High white cell count
  d Lumps around the anus
  e Normal temperature

7 PR bleeding is common in all but ONE of the following:
  a Anal fissure
  b Diverticulitis
  c Bowel malignancy
  d Anal skin tags
  e Angiodysplasia

8 Which of the following is characteristic of a femoral hernia?
  a It points down the leg
  b It points towards the groin
  c Appears above and medial to the pubic tubercle
  d Is more common in men
  e Herniates into a defect called Hesselbach's triangle

9 Which of the following is NOT a predisposing factor for colorectal cancer?
  a Inflammatory bowel disease
  b Irritable bowel disease
  c FAP (familial adenomatous polyposis)
  d Family history
  e Smoking

10 Which is the most common location to find a colorectal cancer?
  a Caecum and ascending colon
  b Transverse colon
  c Descending colon
  d Sigmoid colon
  e Rectum

11 Which is NOT a common characteristic of a perianal abscess?
  a Fluctuant mass
  b Erythematous area
  c Increased white cell count
  d Pain
  e Soft swelling

Answers

SAQs

1 **a** Fresh PR bleeding
Pain on defecation
The patient notices a lump at the anus (sentinel pile)
Typically refuses to permit PR examination due to pain

    b In the midline of the posterior wall of the anal canal.

    c After a vaginal delivery
Inflammatory bowel disease

    d Inflammation around the fissure causes a spasm of the muscle of the internal sphincter.
This spasm affects the inferior rectal artery which compromises the blood supply to the sphincter.

    e Laxatives
Glycerin tri-nitrate (GTN) cream/diltiazem cream
Botulinum toxin injection into anal sphincter

    f Increased incidence of post-operative faecal incontinence

    g Lateral subcutaneous sphincterotomy

Anal fissures are likely to be caused by the passing of hard stools which cause a break in the squamous mucosal lining of the anal canal. Fissures are usually shallow and heal with no complications. However, it is possible for the sphincter to go into spasm reducing the blood supply. This impairs healing and deepens the fissure. Management is either medical with the application of topical creams, or a sphincterotomy can be performed to dilate the sphincter.

2 **a** Weight loss
Change of bowel habit
Fresh or old blood in stool
Malaena/old or digested blood
Family history of rectal cancer
Smoker
Previous history of malignancy

    b Flexible sigmoidoscopy – because it allows direct visualisation of the bowel, and the opportunity to take biopsies.

    c Dukes A – tumour is confined to the bowel wall
Dukes B – tumour extends through the wall of the bowel
Dukes C – lymph node involvement
Dukes D – metastatic deposits

    d Inflammatory bowel disease
Smoking
Age
A diet with large amounts of animal fat and meat and is low in fibre
Family history
FAP
Polyps

    e ➤ Right hemicolectomy – caecal tumours or tumours of the ascending colon.
➤ Left hemicolectomy – tumours of the descending colon.
➤ Abdomino-perineal resection – distal rectal tumours.
➤ Anterior resection – tumours in the lower part of the sigmoid or the proximal part of the rectum.

In patients who present with a change in bowel habit, weight loss, abdominal pain and bloody stools you should be suspicious of a malignancy. CT scans can show bowel strictures and masses but sigmoidoscopy allows direct visualisation of the mucosa and allows biopsies to be taken for histological analysis. Mortality is directly related to the grade of the malignancy (Dukes A–D). There are a number of surgical options depending on the location of the malignancy. Radiotherapy can be used before surgical intervention to decrease local recurrence in rectal cancers. In a Dukes C malignancy chemotherapy may be used as an adjuvant to surgical intervention.

3   **a** Ulcerative colitis
Colorectal cancer
Gastroenteritis
Ischaemic colitis

    b CT scan – shows thickened small bowel loops especially in the terminal ileum
Barium study – wall thickening, cobblestoning, fissures, strictures and fistulas
Magnetic resonance imaging (MRI) – identifies strictures, can differentiate fibrosis from inflammation
Colonoscopy – direct visualisation, allows biopsies

    c Any part of the GI tract from mouth to anus may be affected, however, the most common location is the terminal ileum.

    d Colovesical (between bowel and bladder)
Colovaginal (between colon and vagina)
Enterocutaneous (between the bowel and the skin)

    e Erythema nodosum
Clubbing
Pyoderma gangrenosum

Conjunctivitis
Episcleritis
Ankylosing spondylitis
Sacro-ilitus
Arthritis (in large joints)
Cholelithiasis
Cholangiocarcinoma
f Prednisolone/hydrocortisone – decreases the inflammation
Azathioprine – steroid sparing agent
5-aminosalicylates
Methotrexate
TNF-α inhibitors
g Complications – perforation, fistula, obstruction
To alleviate symptoms when medications have failed
To treat localised terminal ileitis

Crohn's disease is an inflammatory condition which can affect all parts of the GIT, most commonly affecting the terminal ileum. Lesions are not continuous which causes the 'skip lesions' typically associated with the disease. Smoking increases the risk four-fold. Family history is also an important risk factor in developing Crohn's. The medical management of Crohn's focuses on minimising inflammation. Surgery for Crohn's is not curative. Small portions of the worst affected areas may be resected but if too great an area is resected this lead to short gut syndrome.

4 a Enlarged lymph nodes
Lipoma
Varicocele
Saphena varix
b Below the inguinal ligament
Lateral to the pubic tubercle
c Anteriorly – inguinal ligament
Posteriorly – pectineal ligament
Medially – lacunar ligament
Laterally – femoral vein
d It may have become strangulated/incarcerated
e Abdominal pain
Nausea
Vomiting
Abdominal distension
Constipation
f Surgical exploration and reduction, possibly with bowel resection, if the blood supply has been compromised.

Femoral hernias are more common in women than in men. When a hernia becomes strangulated, a portion of bowel protrudes through the weakness as well. This causes an obstruction and leads to obstructive symptoms such as nausea, vomiting and constipation. Often localising signs are not well-defined and abdominal pain tends to be colicky in nature. It requires immediate surgery as if the blood supply to the bowel is compromised it may lead to necrosis, gangrene and perforation.

5 a Bowel cancer
Anal fissure
Diverticular disease
Crohn's disease
Ulcerative colitis

   b Is this the first episode?
Has there been any recent change in bowel habit?
Is it associated with abdominal pain?
Has he noticed any lumps around the anus?
Has he experienced any itching around the anus?
Has he been passing mucus, or just blood?
Any weight loss?

   c Pregnancy
Obesity
Family history
Chronic diarrhoea
Colonic malignancy
Liver disease
Rectal surgery

   d Grade 1 – do not prolapse from anus
Grade 2 – return spontaneously
Grade 3 – require manual return
Grade 4 – prolapsed and irreducible

   e Rubber band ligation
Haemorrhoidectomy
Sclerosant injection
Cryotherapy
Infra-red coagulation
Surgical excision

Haemorrhoids are swollen mucosal pads of vascular cushions. The pads are required for control of bowel movements. They are found at 3, 7 and 11 o'clock positions when looking at the anus in the lithotomy position. They are usually managed medically but can be removed in a haemorrhoidectomy, although this is a very painful procedure.

6 a Ulcerative colitis
   b Uveitis
     Conjunctivitis
     Episcleritis
     Arthritis
     Erythema nodosum
     Pyoderma gangrenosum
     Sacroileitus
     Ankylosing spondylitis
   c Proctitis
   d Ulcerative colitis affecting the entire colon.
   e Goblet cell depletion
     Crypt abscesses
   f In ulcerative colitis, only the colon and rectum are involved whereas in Crohn's, all of the GI tract is affected. Therefore, in Crohn's not all of the affected areas can be removed.

Ulcerative colitis is a form of inflammatory bowel disease. It is more localised than Crohn's disease, being confined to the rectum spreading proximally to the colon but never spreading proximal to the ileocaecal valve. Complications are similar to Crohn's, such as bleeding, perforation and toxic mega-colon. Fistulas are rare in ulcerative colitis. Surgery can be performed to remove the affected portion of the colon. Overall, 20% of patients will require surgical intervention.

7 a A lump or protuberance of skin around the anal verge.
   b Injury/trauma
     Inflammatory lesion
     Prior rectal surgery
   c A skin tag which sits at the site of previous anal injury or pathology such as an anal fissure.
   d Anal fissure
     Anal fistula
     Infection
     Crohn's disease
   e Can cause pruritis and pain, however they are usually asymptomatic.
   f Removed surgically (and biopsied)
     Laser removal of small skin tags
     Cryotherapy
   g In a patient at risk of anal carcinoma (associated with HPV, anal intercourse, smoking, immunosuppression, and inflammatory bowel disease).

Anal skin tags are lumps of skin around the anus which are usually asymptomatic. They may occur at the site of a previous anal injury, infection or operation; however they can form as a result of underlying pathology. Skin tags are associated with anal fissures, fistulas and Crohn's disease. Anal fissures often form sentinel skin tags. They can be excised under LA, however larger or multiple skin tags may require more extensive surgery and may require a GA.

8 a Fluctuant swollen mass
Erythematous area
Painful PR examination
Purulent discharge
Hot
  b Cryptoglandular epithelium (Crypts of Morgagni)
  c *E. coli*
Enterococcus
Bacteriodes
Staphylococcus
  d Crohn's disease
Diabetes
Malignancy
  e Incision and drainage in theatre.
  f It needs to heal by secondary intention to prevent recurrence. If closed a cavity will be created which is likely to become infected again.

Perianal abscesses are infections which start in the crypoglandular tissue lining the anal canal, and then extend to involve the adjacent tissue. Eventually, an abscess forms. Abscesses are usually fairly hard but fluctuant masses. The best treatment option is incision and drainage in theatre as this allows the abscess to be opened, drained and washed out. The cavity is then packed to allow healing from the bottom of the cavity upwards.

9 a Incisional hernia
  b The protrusion of a viscus through the site of a previous operation.
  c Surgical technique
Obesity
Wound infection
Chronic cough
Ischaemia
Diabetes

   d   Strangulation or incarceration
       The neck of the hernia is usually wide preventing any incarceration
       from occurring.
   e   Surgical repair
       Use of a truss

Incisional hernias form at the site of a previous operation where the
muscle join has broken down. This may be because of surgical technique
or patient-related risk factors such as obesity, diabetes, chronic cough or
wound infection. The preferred management option is surgical repair
using a mesh which holds the viscus in. Incisional hernias usually have a
wide neck and, as such, do not usually obstruct or strangulate, although
it is possible.

10 a   Diverticulitis
       Bowel cancer
       Haemorrhoids
       Polyps
       Angiodysplasia
   b   Has there been any weight loss?
       Has there been any change in bowel habit?
       Does she have problems with constipation?
       Has she been told she has diverticular disease?
       Any previous history?
       Any fever?
   c   Diverticulitis
   d   Diverticulae are out-pouchings of the bowel wall. These become
       infected leading to inflammation, pain, and bleeding.
   e   CT scan
   f   IV antibiotics
       IV fluid
       NBM
       Catheter
       Thromboprophylaxis
   g   Abscess formation

Diverticular disease is a disease of the large bowel, usually in the sigmoid.
Diverticulae are out-pouchings of the bowel wall. If these become
infected, it is called diverticulitis. This usually causes an increased white
cell count, fever and tenderness in the LIF. It is treated with broad-
spectrum antibiotics, but severe or recurrent disease may necessitate a
resection of the sigmoid colon.

11 a An abnormal communication between two epithelial surfaces.
   b A fistula between the large bowel and the bladder.
   c From the sigmoid colon to the top of the bladder.
   d Colovaginal (between colon and vagina)
      Enterocutaneous (between the bowel and the skin)
   e Diverticulitis
      Crohn's disease
      Malignancy
      Incomplete separation during embryonic stages
   f CT scan
      Cystoscopy
      Barium enema
      Colonoscopy
      MRI
   g Surgery to remove the fistula and pathological segment of bowel.

A colovesical fistula is an abnormal communication between the epithelium of the large bowel and the epithelium of the bladder. It can be caused by a number of underlying pathologies, it can be congenital, caused by malignancy or be due to complications of previous surgery. Most commonly, it is due to underlying inflammatory processes such as diverticulitis and Crohn's disease. A CT scan may sometimes show the fistula tract. Colonoscopy is useful to exclude malignancy in addition to diagnosis. The only treatment option is surgical intervention.

12 a Roof – internal oblique and transversus abdominis
      Floor – inguinal ligament and lacunar ligament (medial third)
   b Round ligament of the uterus
      Ilioinguinal nerve
   c External spermatic fascia from external oblique
      Internal spermatic fascia from transversalis fascia
      Cremasteric fascia from internal oblique
   d Through a weakness in the posterior wall which is medial to the internal ring.
   e The deep inguinal ring
   f After the hernia has been reduced, ask the patient to cough while pressing over the internal ring. This will stop an indirect hernia but a direct one will come back despite the pressure.
   g Indirect as they may become constricted at the deep inguinal ring.

Inguinal hernias are caused by a weakness in the abdominal muscle wall. Indirect hernias pass through the internal ring and along the inguinal canal. Direct hernias enter directly via a weakness in the posterior wall of the canal. It is possible to differentiate direct from indirect as described above, however, this is usually inaccurate and both types are repaired in the same way. If they become strangulated they become painful, swollen and irreducible and require emergency surgery as the bowel may become ischaemic. Hernias are commonly repaired when asymptomatic to prevent complications.

EMQs

1	E	10	D	19	D
2	B	11	B	20	B
3	A	12	G	21	C
4	G	13	F	22	F
5	F	14	D	23	A
6	A	15	E	24	B
7	H	16	C	25	G
8	G	17	C		
9	B	18	A		

MCQs

1 a and c – An anal fissure is a very painful condition with patients also presenting with a sentinel pile and discharge. Treatment is with stool softeners, and the use of GTN or diltiazem cream prior to surgical intervention if these fail.

2 b – Crohn's disease affects the bowel from the mouth to the anus, with associated systemic features. It also occurs in skip lesions, and affects the full thickness of the bowel.

3 b – Colovesical fistulae are three times more common in women than men.

4 d – There are several extra-intestinal signs of inflammatory bowel disease including erythema nodosum, clubbing, pyoderma gangrenosum, conjunctivitis, episcleritis, ankylosing spondylitis, sacro-ilitus, arthritis (in large joints), cholelithiasis, and cholangiocarcinoma.

5 b – Strangulation is least common in incisional hernias due to the larger size of the hernia orifice.

6 c – Haemorrhoids do not cause a raised white cell count.

7 d – Anal skin tags are covered with stratified squamous epithelium, therefore, they do not bleed.

8 a – Femoral hernias are protrusions through the femoral canal into the femoral triangle. They are, therefore, lateral to the pubic tubercle and point down the leg.

9 b – Irritable bowel disease is not a risk factor of colorectal cancer.

10 e – Bowel cancer most commonly occurs in the rectum.

11 e – A perianal abscess presents with a painful, red, swollen, warm area around the anus, which typically requires incision and drainage.

Chapter 3

Upper GI surgery

Wai Kien Ng

SAQs

1 A 55-year-old caucasian male with a long-standing history of dyspepsia was seen in A&E complaining of retrosternal discomfort. Based on his medical history you think that he has gastro-oesophageal reflux disease (GORD).

 a Give two risk factors for GORD. (2 marks)
 b Although you suspect that this is a likely case of GORD, what other acute medical condition must you exclude in this patient? (1 mark)
 c Having done the relevant investigations, you are satisfied that this patient is medically safe to be discharged home with outpatient follow-up. Give two further tests you could use to diagnose this condition. (2 marks)
 d Following the above investigations, histology results were consistent with Barrett's oesophagus. What is Barrett's oesophagus? (2 marks)
 e Besides Barrett's oesophagus, give two other complications of GORD. (2 marks)
 f Why is it important to follow up patients with Barrett's oesophagus? (1 mark)
 g Give two management options available to this patient. (2 marks)

2 A 42-year-old lady presents with a sudden onset of epigastric pain radiating to the back. She is vomiting, and clearly in a lot of pain. You are the junior doctor on-call, and suspect she has acute pancreatitis.

 a List two other differential diagnoses. (2 marks)
 b On examination, this lady is tachycardic, pale and clammy. You also find that she has some bluish discoloration around her umbilicus. Name this sign. (1 mark)
 c Give three ways in which you would investigate this patient further. (3 marks)
 d How would you manage this patient initially? (2 marks)
 e List two scoring systems used to assess the severity of acute pancreatitis. (2 marks)
 f List two complications of acute pancreatitis. (2 marks)
 g Give two risk factors for developing acute pancreatitis. (2 marks)

3 A 55-year-old man presents with a 4-week history of malaise, weight loss and pruritus.

    a Give two further questions you would ask to try to establish a diagnosis. (2 marks)

    b On examination, he is jaundiced and there is a palpable mass in the left supraclavicular fossa. What is the name given to this lump and what is its significance? (2 marks)

    c You can also feel a palpable gallbladder. What is Courvoisier's law? (1 mark)

    d You suspect that this man may have an underlying malignancy, most likely to be pancreatic in origin. Give two ways in which you would investigate this further. (2 marks)

    e He was found to have a 2 cm lesion in the head of the pancreas, with regional lymph node involvement, metastases to the liver and intraperitoneal seedings. What is his tumour, node, metastasis (TNM) staging? (2 marks)

    f Briefly outline Whipple's procedure. (2 marks)

4 A 62-year-old lady from China was in the UK to visit her son who is a student at a local university. During this visit, she was feeling unwell and was having dyspepsia, dysphagia and vomiting. As her symptoms did not settle, she was seen by a GP who has referred her to the hospital.

    a Give three risk factors for developing gastric cancer. (3 marks)

    b Name two ways in which gastric tumours spread. (2 marks)

    c List three physical signs you may find if the disease is in its advanced stages. (3 marks)

    d Give three investigations which would be useful in this case. (3 marks)

    e Which healthcare professionals would you expect to find in upper GI multi-disciplinary team (MDT) meetings? (2 marks)

5 A 50-year-old lady was admitted with a 6 hour history of upper abdominal pain which is getting worse. The pain started after she ate a big meal at a friend's house. She had previous similar episodes of abdominal pain before.

    a Give three risk factors for developing cholecystitis. (3 marks)

    b Apart from cholecystitis list two further differential diagnoses. (2 marks)

    c Give three ways in which you will manage a patient with acute cholecystitis. (3 marks)

    d What is the radiological investigation that you would request initially for this patient, and why? (2 marks)

    e Explain Murphy's sign. (2 marks)

f Give three possible complications that can arise from acute cholecystitis. (3 marks)

6 A 54-year-old lady presented with intermittent RUQ pain. It started about 2 hours after eating fish and chips. She is also tachycardic and has been sick in the last hour. She is now complaining of pleuritic pain.
a Give two risk factors for developing gallstones. (2 marks)
b Name two possible components of a gallstone. (2 marks)
c Give three aspects of your initial management plan. (3 marks)
d Upon further questioning, she told you that she had a similar episode a fortnight ago. She assumed that it was a case of indigestion and did not seek medical advice on that occasion. What is the initial investigation of choice? (1 mark)
e She also had an abdominal X-ray which did not reveal any stones. She was admitted for further observation. During the night, she was pyrexial and was having rigors. What is likely to have happened to cause these new symptoms? (1 mark)
f What antibiotics would you use to treat this lady? (1 mark)

7 A 37-year-old man was referred by his GP after experiencing two episodes of coffee ground vomiting. He was recently discharged from hospital following an operation on a fractured femur sustained during a road traffic accident (RTA). On admission, his BP was 132/74, pulse was 82 bpm.
a List three further pieces of information you would like to elicit to help you to look for the possible cause and source of bleeding. (3 marks)
b As you are sending off the bloods, the nurse informs you that this patient's BP is now 98/62, and pulse 58 bpm. Give two aspects of management you should initiate urgently. (2 marks)
c The on-call surgeon was informed and an endoscopy was carried out. Multiple superficial bleeding ulcers were found. Adrenaline was injected to achieve haemostasis. How does adrenaline exert this effect? (2 marks)
d What other materials/substance can be used to achieve haemostasis in this situation? (1 mark)
e He was haemodynamically stable and was returned to the ward after the endoscopy. What medication should he be started on? (1 mark)
f This patient was taking his wife's rheumatoid arthritis medication (diclofenac) for pain relief after the fractured femur operation. How should you advise this patient prior to discharge? (2 marks)

8 Michael, a 56-year-old business executive has presented today with pain in his stomach that occurs typically after meals. In the past, he has tried some over the counter (OTC) medications which have offered him some relief.

    a Explain the pathophysiology of gastric ulcers. (2 marks)

    b Give three risk factors for developing gastric ulcers. (3 marks)

    c Name two possible complications of gastric ulcer disease. (2 marks)

    d He was referred for an urgent upper GI endoscopy because of his age. What are the alarm symptoms that would also prompt an urgent upper GI referral? (2 marks)

    e A few months later, Michael is still complaining of the same pain. He was referred to an upper GI surgeon for consideration of surgery. What procedure may be done for gastric ulceration? (2 marks)

9 Alan, a 60-year-old man was seen in A&E with generalised abdominal tenderness. On examination, his abdomen is rigid and board-like. He is lying still and barely moves when you enter the examination room. You also notice that he is taking shallow breaths.

    a He has had a cannula inserted and bloods sent in A&E. Give three aspects of his management you would initiate next. (3 marks)

    b What investigations should you request now and why? (2 marks)

    c Your investigations show that this patient has a perforation. What management does he now require? (1 mark)

    d List two other complications of duodenal ulcer. (2 marks)

    e Other than OGD give two investigations you would request to investigate a patient with suspected peptic ulcer disease. (2 marks)

    f Why is endoscopy the preferred investigation of choice? (2 marks)

10 A 54-year-old man was admitted with a 5-month history of weight loss and pain in the RUQ. On examination, an enlarged and irregular liver was felt 2 cm below the ribcage. He also tells you that he is an ex-IV drug user.

    a What other signs of chronic liver disease would you look out for? Name three. (3 marks)

    b List two risk factors for developing hepatocellular carcinoma (HCC). (2 marks)

    c You had a needle stick injury while taking blood from this patient. Assuming that he is positive for Hepatitis B, C and HIV, what is the risk of being infected with Hepatitis B, C, and HIV respectively? (3 marks)

d   Name a tumour marker that can be used to monitor the
     progress of the disease.   (1 mark)
e   How can HCC be prevented?   (2 marks)

EMQs

Match the following descriptions:
A Krukenberg tumour
B Virchow's nodes
C Thrombophlebitis migrans
D Sister Mary Joseph nodes
E Curling's ulcer
F Chovstek's sign
G Cushing's ulcer
H Grey Turner's sign
I Cullen's sign

1 An umbilical nodule due to intra-abdominal malignancy.
2 A palpable node in the left supraclavicular fossa.
3 Discoloration in periumbilical area.
4 Stress ulcer in the stomach, resulting from neurosurgery.
5 Transcoelemic spread to the ovaries in females.
6 Alternating inflammation of the veins.
7 Discoloration around the flanks.
8 Stress ulcer in the stomach as a result of severe burns.

Match the following staging system with the disease:
A Acute pancreatitis
B Acute cholecystitis
C Acute appendicitis
D Diverticulitis
E Prostate cancer
F Bladder cancer
G Colorectal cancer
H Oesophageal cancer
I Child-Pugh classification

9   Dukes' classification.
10 Modified Glasgow criteria.
11 Alvarado score.
12 Gleason grading.
13 End-stage liver disease.

Match the following:
A Chronic pancreatitis
B Acute pancreatitis
C Biliary colic
D Oesophageal atresia
E Intussusception
F GORD
G Acute appendicitis

14 A newborn was treated for aspiration pneumonia after regurgitating his feed.
15 Feeling of retrosternal discomfort after eating.
16 Nausea, vomiting, colicky RUQ pain radiating to the shoulder blades.
17 Abdominal pain post-endoscopic retrograde cholangiopancreatography (ERCP).
18 PR bleeding that looks like redcurrant jelly.

Which of the following are associated?
A Hepatitis B
B Crohn's disease
C Pernicious anaemia
D Achalasia
E Schistosomiasis

19 Bladder cancer.
20 Hepatocellular carcinoma.
21 Stomach cancer.
22 Colorectal cancer.
23 Oesophageal cancer.

Match the diagnosis with the description:
A Cholelithiasis
B Cholecystitis
C Gallbladder empyema
D Ascending cholangitis
E Cholangiocarcinoma
F Gallstone ileus

24 A patient with previous recurrent cholecystitis presenting with a swinging pyrexia.
25 Characterised by the triad of RUQ pain, jaundice, and fever with rigors.
26 Intermittent RUQ pain following fatty meals.
27 A painless palpable gallbladder in a patient with jaundice.
28 Small bowel obstruction occurring due to an occlusion at the ileocaecal valve.

MCQs

1 A 54-year-old lady was admitted with acute cholecystitis. What is the most appropriate initial treatment?
a   Open cholecystectomy
b   Laparoscopic cholecystectomy
c   Incision and drainage
d   Laparotomy and proceed
e   None of the above

2 A 79-year-old man was admitted with nausea, abdominal distension and reported that he had not opened his bowels for a few days. Abdominal X-ray showed features of ileus. What is the most appropriate initial management?
a   Surgery
b   Antibiotic therapy
c   NBM, IV fluids and nasogastric (NG) tube
d   Arrange for an urgent CT scan

3 Which of the enzymes below is the most sensitive and specific for pancreatitis?
a   Serum lactate dehydrongenase (LDH)
b   Serum aspartate transaminase (AST)
c   Serum amylase
d   Serum lipase
e   Serum triptase

4 An indirect inguinal hernia is located:
a   Lateral to the inferior epigastric artery
b   Medial to the inferior epigastric artery
c   Medial to the superior epigastric artery
d   Lateral to the superior epigastric artery

5 Gastric carcinoma is associated with:
a   Type A blood group
b   Type B blood group
c   Type O blood group
d   Type AB blood group
e   All of the above

6 Complications/side-effects of peptic ulcer surgery include:
   a Diarrhoea
   b Dumping syndrome
   c Early satiety
   d Anaemia
   e All of the above

7 Which of the below is not associated with oesophageal carcinoma?
   a Osler–Weber–Rendu syndrome
   b Plummer–Vinson syndrome
   c Barrett's oesophagus
   d Paterson–Brown–Kelly syndrome
   e None of the above

8 Modified Glasgow criteria are calculated from the following except:
   a Albumin
   b Calcium
   c Age
   d Creatinine
   e White cell count

9 Mr Smith was referred by his GP because he was complaining of frequent dyspepsia. What are the alarm features of dyspepsia that would prompt a referral for an urgent endoscopy?
   a Iron deficiency anaemia
   b Dysphagia
   c Weight loss and anorexia
   d Recent onset of progressive symptoms
   e All of the above

10 Medications used in the treatment of GORD include:
   a Magnesium trisilicate mixture
   b Lansoprazole
   c Metoclopramide
   d Alginates
   e All of the above

Answers

SAQs

1 a Hiatus hernia
Increased intra-abdominal pressure (obesity, pregnancy)
Smoking
Alcohol
Big meals
Caffeine

    b MI

    c Barium meal
OGD
CLO test for *H. pylori*

    d Barrett's oesophagus is the change from one differentiated cell type into another differentiated cell type in the lower end of the oesophagus, from squamous cell to columnar cell.

    e Oesophagitis
Respiratory complications such as pneumonia and interstitial lung disease
Anaemia
Oesophageal stricture

    f There is a risk of developing carcinoma of the oesophagus, although this risk is less than 1% per year.

    g Medical management with proton pump inhibitors (PPIs)
Surgical management (e.g. fundoplication, vagotomy)
Lifestyle modification (smaller frequent meals, smoking cessation, alcohol and caffeine cessation, weight loss, avoid eating before bedtime)

Barrett's oesophagus is the change from squamous to columnar cells at the lower end of the oesophagus due to persistent GORD. It typically presents with heartburn, acid brash, and odynophagia, and is diagnosed endoscopically. Treatment is commonly through the use of PPIs and lifestyle changes, with regular surveillance endoscopy.

2 a Cholecystitis
Biliary colic
Cholangitis
Perforated peptic ulcer
Ruptured AAA

Pyelonephritis
MI

b   Cullen's sign

c   Blood tests (FBC, U+Es, LFTs, Ca, amylase levels, CRP, glucose, albumin)
Arterial blood gas
Urinalysis (pregnancy test, urine dip, MC&S)
Erect chest X-ray, abdominal X-ray

d   IV fluids
Urinary catheter to monitor output
Analgesia
Thromboprophylaxis
NBM
Antiemetics
NG tube if vomiting

e   Modified Glasgow criteria
Ranson criteria
APACHE II

f   Early complication (shock, acute respiratory distress syndrome (ARDS), acute renal failure, disseminated intravascular coagulation (DIC), intra-abdominal sepsis)
Late complications (abscess formation, pseudocyst, necrosis)

g   Gallstones
Alcohol
Trauma
Drug induced (steroids, azathioprine)
Infections (mumps, measles), parasitic infections (Ascaris lumbricoides, Clonorchis sinensis)
Congenital anomalies (pancreas divisum/annular pancreas)

Acute pancreatitis typically presents with a sudden onset of epigastric pain which radiates to the tip of the scapula. Treatment is mainly supportive with aggressive rehydration, analgesia, and monitoring of urine output. The pancreas should also be rested, by keeping the patient NBM.

3 a   Duration of symptoms
Change in skin, stool and urine colour
Lifestyle questions (alcohol, smoking, diet, exercise)
Any previous history of pancreatitis, cholecystitis, biliary colic
Family history of cancer

b   Virchow's node
Its presence may signify the presence of gastric cancer

c   A palpable gallbladder in the presence of painless jaundice is unlikely to be due to gallstones.

d Blood tests (FBC, U+Es, LFTs, amylase, calcium, CA19-9)
Radiology (ultrasound scan (USS) abdomen, CT scan)
MRCP+/- ERCP

e T1N1M1

f Whipple's procedure is the resection of the head of the pancreas, duodenum, upper jejunum, the distal half of the stomach, gallbladder, and lower half of the CBD along with the regional lymph nodes. Then a cholecystojejunostomy, gastrojejunostomy and pancreaticojejunostomy are performed.

Pancreatic cancer has a very poor prognosis, with a 5-year survival of only 5%. They are most commonly adenocarcinoma and often present late as it is typically asymptomatic. Patients may, however, present with pain, loss of appetite, obstructive jaundice, weight loss, and diabetes.

4   **a** Diet (salted fish, preserved meat nitrates)
Familial
H. pylori
Pernicious anaemia
Blood group A
Chronic atrophic gastritis
Smoking

b Local (direct invasion into adjacent structures)
Lymphatic spread as in metastases

c Virchow's node – Troisier's sign (enlarged supraclavicular lymph node on the left side)
Sister Mary Joseph nodules (periumbilical metastases)
Ascites
Hepatomegaly
Jaundice
Paraneoplastic syndromes (acanthosis nigricans, dermatomyositis)

d Bloods (FBC, U+Es, LFTs, calcium profile, tumour markers)
OGD and biopsies
CT/MRI for staging
Positron emission tomography (PET) scan

e Upper GI surgeons
Gastroenterologist
Radiologist
Pathologist
Specialist nurse
Oncologist
Palliative care team

Gastric cancer typically presents initially with vague symptoms of abdominal discomfort, indigestion, and loss of appetite, and may progress to weight loss, bleeding, and dysphagia. It is more common in patients who eat smoked food, have *H. pylori*, and smoke.

5   **a**   Increasing age
Female sex
Obesity
Pregnancy
Haemolytic anaemia

     b   Pancreatitis
Biliary colic
Perforated duodenal/peptic ulcer
AAA
MI
Lower lobe pneumonia

     c   NBM
IV fluids
Analgesia
Antibiotics

     d   Abdominal ultrasound
Ultrasound is able to detect 90% of gallstones. In addition, ultrasonography allows measurement of the CBD, and thickness of the gallbladder.

     e   On palpation of the RUQ, at the tip of the 9th costal cartilage, pain is elicited when the patient breathes in, as the inflamed gallbladder hits the fingers.
For this to be truly positive, it should also be performed on the left and found negative.

     f   Pancreatitis
Perforation
Ascending cholangitis
Gallbladder empyema

Cholecystitis is due to an infection in the gallbladder resulting in a distended oedematous gallbladder. This requires treatment with antibiotics, and imaging of the biliary tree to ensure the CBD is clear prior to cholecystectomy. Operative intervention is best done 6 weeks post-inflammation; however, this is not always possible due to the high percentage of patients with recurrent or chronic disease.

6 a Fat
Female
Fertile
Forty
Fair
b Bile salts
Cholesterol
Calcium carbonate
Bilirubin
c NBM
Establish venous access + IV fluids
Bloods including FBC, U+E, LFT's, CRP
Analgesia
ECG (to rule out MI).
d Ultrasound of the abdomen
e Ascending cholangitis
f Co-amoxiclav and metronidazole

Cholelithiasis typically presents as colicky pain in the RUQ which often radiates to the back after a fatty meal. Patients may also present with nausea, vomiting and sweating. Bloods should be sent to ensure there is no infection or obstruction to the biliary tree. These patients should undergo elective laparoscopic cholecystectomy.

7 a Clotting abnormalities
Alcohol consumption (e.g. bleeding varices)
Recent trauma/illness
Previous GI bleed
Dyspepsia
Previous peptic/duodenal ulcer
Medications (warfarin, aspirin, clopidogrel)
b Fluid resus (500 ml of gelofusin stat to bring the BP up)
Ensure good IV access (two large bore cannulae antecubitally)
Give IV PPI
Call for help and inform endoscopy as this patient may need urgent endoscopy to look for and to stop the source of bleeding.
c Adrenaline is a vasoactive agent. It induces vasoconstriction and hence decreases blood flow to the area. This allows the haemostatic mechanism to work effectively.
d Fibrin glue
Sclerosants (e.g. ethanol)
Laser phototherapy
Direct pressure
Thermal therapy

  e PPIs initially IV
  f Advise him to stop taking medication that is not prescribed for him.
   Change to another type of analgesia
   Follow up with his GP
   Continue taking his PPIs

There are several causes of haematemesis including Mallory-Weiss tear, oesophageal varices, gastric ulcers, and gastric cancer. It is a surgical emergency as patients will often lose considerable amounts of blood into the bowel, and may become shocked. Endoscopic assessment to control the bleeding may be required rapidly.

8 a Gastric ulcers develop when there is an over-production of HCl and pepsin compared to mucous and bicarbonate. This leads to the acid eroding the stomach lining causing ulceration.
  b *H. pylori*
   Non-steroidal anti-inflammatory drugs (NSAIDs)
   Zollinger–Ellison syndrome (rare)
   Chemotherapeutic agents
   Bisphosphonates
   Smoking
   Stress (Curling's ulcer)
  c Perforation
   Bleeding
   Peritonitis
   Subphrenic abscess
   Gastric cancer
  d Anaemia
   Weight loss
   Malaena/haematemesis
   Dysphagia
   Worsening symptoms
  e Highly selective vagotomy – the vagus nerve is denervated only where it supplies the stomach and lower oesophagus. This operation does not affect gastric emptying and the success of this operation is greatly dependent on the surgeon. It is rarely done now due to the use of PPIs.

Patients presenting with alarm symptoms should be referred for an urgent upper GI endoscopy. In most cases, they are managed medically, however a small group of patients may not respond or tolerate medical treatment and hence may require surgery.

9 a IV fluids
        Keep NBM
        Urinary catheter
        Oxygen
        Analgesia
        Erect chest X-ray and abdominal X-ray
   b Erect chest X-ray – to look for free air under diaphragm which may signify a perforation of a viscus
        Abdominal X-ray – to look for any signs of obstruction
   c Laparotomy and proceed
   d Malignancy
        Pyloric obstruction
        Bleeding
        Subphrenic abscess
        Subdiaphragmatic abscess
   e CLO test
        Barium meal
        Urea breath test
        Blood test for *H. pylori*/stool test for *H. pylori*
   f It is both a diagnostic and therapeutic investigation.
        It can be used to get tissue samples for biopsy and achieve haemostasis in bleeding ulcers if needed.

Duodenal ulcer is more common than gastric ulcer. It is associated with *H. pylori*, NSAIDs and aspirin use, especially in the elderly. Patients should be advised to avoid foods that worsen their symptoms, take small frequent meals, stop smoking, decrease alcohol consumption and lifestyle modifications including stress management and weight control. PPI's are highly effective treatments, and have dramatically decreased the number of patients requiring surgical intervention.

10 a Spider naevi
        Gynaecomastia
        Caput medusa
        Dupuytren's contracture
        Clubbing
        Palmar erythema
        Ascites
   b Viral hepatitis (Hepatitis B or C)
        Cirrhosis
        Haemochromotosis
        Aflatoxins

c   Hepatitis B – 30%
     Hepatitis C – 3%
     HIV – 0.3%
d   Alpha feto protein.
e   Hepatitis B vaccinations
     Practising safe sex
     Do not share needles
     Reducing alcohol intake
     Screening of blood products

HCC is a primary malignancy of the liver and it primarily affects patients with underlying cirrhosis and chronic liver disease. The incidence is highest in Africa and Asia mainly in part due to the endemic Hepatitis B and C in these regions. Increasing alcohol abuse in western countries is leading to a rise in the frequency of alcoholic liver disease and subsequently cirrhosis and HCC.

EMQs

1	D	11	C	21	C
2	B	12	E	22	B
3	I	13	I	23	D
4	G	14	D	24	B
5	A	15	F	25	D
6	C	16	C	26	A
7	H	17	B	27	E
8	E	18	E	28	F
9	G	19	E		
10	A	20	A		

MCQs

1   e – In acute cholecystitis, treatment is initially conservative. Surgical intervention is generally not indicated unless there is evidence that the gallbladder has perforated. Most surgeons prefer to wait for 6–8 weeks before operating to allow the inflammation to settle.

2   c – It is important to correct any electrolyte imbalance and to rehydrate the patient. Vomiting, poor appetite and decreased oral intake can make the patient very dehydrated.

3   d – Serum amylase levels begin to fall within the first 24–48 hours. A patient with pancreatitis may have a normal amylase level. Serum lipase is more sensitive and specific for pancreatitis.

4   a – An indirect inguinal hernia lies lateral to the inferior epigastric artery, whereas a direct inguinal hernia lies medially.

5   a – Gastric carcinoma is more commonly associated with blood group A than any other blood groups.

6   e – Elective peptic ulcer surgery is not commonly performed nowadays due to the effective medical therapy available to treat peptic ulcers. However, all of the above may be a complication or side effect of peptic ulcer surgery.

7   a – Plummer–Vinson syndrome and Paterson–Brown–Kelly syndrome are the same syndrome. Barrett's oesophagus increases a person's risk of developing oesophageal carcinoma. Osler–Weber–Rendu syndrome causes telangiectasia of the skin and mucous membranes and may be associated with iron deficiency anaemia as a result of chronic blood loss from the GIT.

8   d – Modified Glasgow criteria are used to predict the severity of pancreatitis. Criteria include pO_2, age, white cell count, calcium levels, urea levels, enzymes (alkaline transaminase/AST/LDH), albumin and blood glucose level.

9   e – Any patient presenting with alarm features/if the patient is >55 years old should be referred for urgent endoscopy.

10 e – All of the above medications can be used to treat GORD. Gaviscon (an alginate) is frequently used to provide relief from symptoms of GORD, however, PPI's are a more common long term alternative.

Chapter 4

Vascular surgery

Georgina Riddiough

SAQs

1 A 60-year-old man attends A&E complaining of acute onset abdominal pain radiating to the back. He has a past medical history of hypertension and hypercholesterolaemia. His BP is 80/50 and heart rate is 130 regular. On examination, you notice bilateral bruising in the flanks.
 a Please list the most likely diagnosis and three further differential diagnoses? (4 marks)
 b List three risk factors for developing this condition. (3 marks)
 c List two radiological investigations that can be used to assess this condition. (3 marks)
 d This gentleman is tall and thin and you notice he has long, thin fingers. What underlying diagnosis do you suspect? (1 mark)

2 A 60-year-old man attends clinic and complains of pain in both calves which comes on after he has walked around 400 metres. He is unable to walk off the pain which is relieved only by rest.
 a What is the most likely diagnosis? (1 mark)
 b Name three conditions you would specifically ask him about in his past medical history. (3 marks)
 c What is the ankle brachial pressure index (ABPI) and how is it calculated? (2 marks)
 d In what group of patients may ABPI be falsely elevated? (1 mark)
 e Give three aspects of lifestyle advice you would give this gentleman. (3 marks)

3 A 75-year-old woman with a past medical history of atrial fibrillation and hypertension is seen by you in A&E with an acutely painful right leg. On examination she is unable to move her toes and has reduced sensation. You suspect acute limb ischaemia.
 a What is the most likely source of embolus in this patient? (1 mark)
 b What are the six cardinal features of acute limb ischaemia? (3 marks)
 c What medical treatment would you commence immediately, and how would you monitor this? (2 marks)

d   What are the two main definitive treatment options for
this condition?   (2 marks)

e   Assuming there are no contraindications, name two
drugs this patient would ideally be discharged home with. (2 marks)

f   Embolism is not always due to an arterial embolus.
Name two other forms of embolism.   (2 marks)

4   A 63-year-old gentleman attends A&E with right-sided facial weakness
and an associated right-sided hemiparesis and hemisensory loss. He is also
dysphasic. In your initial assessment of the patient you request an urgent
CT head scan which rules out intracranial haemorrhage and shows no
other gross abnormalities, other than cerebral atrophy consistent with
the patient's age. You make the diagnosis of an ischaemic stroke. On
examination, he has loud carotid bruits bilaterally and an obvious left
sided hemianopia.

a   According to the Oxford Classification of Stroke what
type of stroke has this man had?   (1 mark)

b   Are carotid bruits a reliable guide to the severity of
carotid artery stenosis? Justify your answer.   (2 marks)

c   Why would an ECG be a useful investigation in this
patient?   (1 mark)

d   This patient has a carotid duplex scan showing a stenosis
of 75% in both internal carotid arteries. What specific
surgical procedure should this gentleman undergo?   (2 marks)

e   Describe four steps in the long term medical
management of this patient.   (4 marks)

5   You see an elderly lady in clinic with a history of diabetes mellitus. She
describes walking as 'like walking on clouds' and on examination, you
notice a large erythematous and infected ulcer over the base of the first
metacarpal on the right foot.

a   List three signs you may notice in the leg/foot of a
patient with diabetes mellitus.   (3 marks)

b   You decide to admit this lady for IV antibiotics. Name
two antibiotics you would prescribe.   (2 marks)

c   List four pieces of advice you would give this lady
upon discharge to try to reduce the risk of further foot
infections.   (4 marks)

d   The lady comes back to clinic and on questioning
it seems she has not followed your advice. On
examination, her right foot is grossly abnormal in shape.
What is the name given to this condition?   (1 mark)

6 A 65-year-old lady is referred to you in clinic with a long-standing ulcer above the medial malleolus on the left. You suspect that this lady has venous hypertension and that the ulcer is venous in origin. You also notice some varicose veins on the posterior aspect of her calf.

    a Name four other signs of chronic venous disease you would look for on examination of this patient. (4 marks)

    b In what venous system are this patient's varicosities found? (1 mark)

    c State one investigation you would request and why. (2 marks)

    d Describe briefly the pathophysiology of venous hypertension. (2 marks)

    e Six months later, you review this lady again in clinic and notice that the ulcer has developed a rolled pearly edge. You strongly suspect malignant change and send a biopsy of tissue to confirm the diagnosis. What is the name given to this condition? (1 mark)

7 A 35-year-old lady was admitted with acute appendicitis. Post-operatively you notice that she has left calf swelling. Examination reveals left calf tenderness and passive dorsiflexion of the left foot induces pain.

    a List two differential diagnoses. (2 marks)

    b Give one blood test you could request to aid your diagnosis, and explain why it would not be useful in this patient. (2 marks)

    c List three prophylactic measures that can help reduce the frequency of thromboembolic events in surgical patients. (3 marks)

    d Outline your definitive management plan for this patient, stating exactly how long you would treat the patient. (4 marks)

8 A 27-year-old lady attends the A&E department. She is 17-weeks pregnant and complains of an acutely painful, swollen and red right calf. You suspect a DVT and commence appropriate treatment.

    a List four risk factors for DVT. (4 marks)

    b What is the name of the probability scoring system used for DVTs? (1 mark)

    c On examination, give three signs you would be looking for other than Homan's sign. (3 marks)

    d What is Homan's sign? (1 mark)

    e What investigation would you request in order to confirm your diagnosis? (1 mark)

9 A 35-year-old lady is referred to you in clinic from her GP. She has a past medical history of rheumatoid arthritis. She reports her fingers change colour when she is cold; they turn white initially and then blue and red. This is also associated with some pain in the tips of her fingers.

   a What is the diagnosis? (1 mark)

   b List two other conditions apart from rheumatoid arthritis which may be associated with this. (2 marks)

   c Give two further signs that may be seen in the hands in this patient. (2 marks)

   d What two pieces of advice would you give this lady? (2 marks)

   e Suggest two investigations that may aid you in the diagnosis of this condition. (2 marks)

   f Name one drug that could be used in the management of this condition. (1 mark)

10 You attend clinic with a renal transplant consultant who wishes to question you further about transplantation.

   a What are the three commonest causes of end stage renal failure in the United Kingdom? (3 marks)

   b What is the definition of end stage renal failure? (1 mark)

   c List three important investigations to carry out in the pre-operative work up of any transplant patient. (3 marks)

   d Name one commonly used immunosuppressant. (1 mark)

   e List two key side effects of immunosuppression. (2 marks)

EMQs

Select from the list the most appropriate diagnosis.

A Berry aneursym
B Mycotic aneurysm
C Dissecting aneurysm
D False aneurysm
E Arteriovenous aneurysm
F Ruptured AAA
G Popliteal aneurysm

1 A 50-year-old man with polycystic kidney disease presents to the A&E department with sudden onset occipital headache and collapse. On examination, he has a positive Kernig's sign.

2 A 38-year-old woman with chronic renal failure had a brachiocephalic fistula created about 1 month ago. She has noticed a pulsatile lump over the skin incision where the fistula was created.

3 A 64-year-old man in the resuscitation bay in A&E requires urgent surgical review. He was admitted with sudden onset abdominal pain and has bilateral bruising in his flanks.

4 A 25-year-old female with a history of IV drug use has come to hospital complaining of a painful, pulsatile lump in her groin.

5 A 45-year-old man with Marfan's syndrome attends A&E with sudden tearing chest pain radiating to between his scapula. On examination, he has unequal pulses in his upper limbs.

Select the most appropriate management for the cases listed below:

A Best medical therapy
B Surgical embolectomy
C Angioplasty
D Amputation
E Femoral–popliteal bypass

6 You see a diabetic patient in clinic who has recently developed cramping pains in his calves on exertion. These come on after walking ~366 metres. You ask the vascular nurses to do ABPIs. Right leg ABPI = 0.85. Left leg APBI = 0.91.

7 A 72-year-old man is admitted under the general surgeons with acute, severe pain in his right leg associated with numbness and difficulty moving his toes. On examination, the foot is cold and pale with absent pulses.

8 An elderly lady is seen in clinic with a history of pain in her left leg worse at night. To relieve the pain she hangs her leg out of bed. On examination, she has a small punched-out ulcer on the base of her heel. She has an angiogram which demonstrates a short section of stenosis in the superficial femoral artery at the level of the adductor canal with good run off into distal vessels.

9 An elderly man has gangrene in his right foot secondary to critical limb ischaemia. An angiogram demonstrates an AAA, diameter 4.5 cm and severe stenosis in his superficial femoral artery with poor distal circulation. He has been on IV antibiotics which are not improving the infection.

10 A 45-year-old gentleman who has smoked heavily for 30 years attends clinic with a history of buttock and thigh pain on walking. You suspect intermittent claudication and decide to perform an angiogram which reveals a short stenosis within the common femoral artery.

Select the most appropriate answer for each question; each answer may be used once, more than once or not at all.

A Short saphenous vein
B Long saphenous vein
C Sural nerve
D Popliteal vein
E Saphenous nerve
F Dorsal venous arch
G Saphenofemoral junction
H Ulnar nerve
I None of the above

11 Passes anterior to the medial malleolus.
12 Runs anterior to the lateral malleolus.
13 Accompanies the short saphenous vein.
14 A branch of the tibial nerve.
15 A patient has varicosities which ascend the medical aspect of her leg to the inside of her groin.

Please match the diagnosis with the description below.

A Short saphenous system varicosities
B Long saphenous system varicosities
C Venous ulcer
D Chronic venous disease
E Arterial ulcer
F Neuropathic ulcer
G Saphena varix
H Femoral hernia

16 A 66-year-old lady attends vascular clinic with varicose veins that appear on the posterior aspect of her right leg and ascend to the popliteal fossa.
17 A patient has a shallow ulcer over the medial malleolus.
18 A patient has a blackened, necrotic ulcer on the base of their left heel.
19 A patient has a punched out ulcer over the base of the second metatarsal.
20 A 72-year-old gentleman attends his local GP complaining of a swelling in his groin, it transmits a cough impulse and has a bluish tinge. It reduces in size when he lies down.

Select the most appropriate answer from the list below for the following statements and scenarios about transplantation.

A Graft vs. host disease
B Post-transplant lymphoproliferative disorder
C Kaposi's sarcoma
D Squamous cell carcinoma
E Tacrolimus
F Azathioprine
G Allograft
H Xenograft
I Autograft

21 Tissue is transferred between genetically dissimilar individuals.
22 Commonly used immunosuppressive drug which is a calcineurin inhibitor.
23 Skin cancer which may also occur in patients with acquired immunodeficiency syndrome (AIDS).
24 A patient who previously underwent a bone marrow transplant develops fever, weight loss, rash and hepatosplenomegaly.
25 Tissue is transferred between different species.

MCQs

1 Which of the following is not a type of aneurysm?
  a   Saccular
  b   Fusiform
  c   Dissecting
  d   Mycotic
  e   Real

2 Which of the following is not a risk factor for peripheral vascular disease (PVD)?
  a   Smoking
  b   Age
  c   Exercise
  d   Hyperlipidaemia
  e   Diabetes mellitus

3 Which of the following is not a branch of the abdominal aorta?
  a   Renal arteries
  b   Vertebral arteries
  c   Inferior phrenic arteries
  d   Suprarenal arteries
  e   Coeliac trunk

4 Which of the following is not a recognised treatment for Raynaud's syndrome?
  a   Avoid common triggers
  b   Prostaglandin analogues
  c   Noradrenaline
  d   Calcium channel blockers
  e   Smoking cessation

5 Which of the following signs and symptoms are not associated with acute limb ischaemia?
  a   Pain
  b   Pallor
  c   Cold
  d   Inflammation
  e   Pulseless

6 Which of the following viruses are tested for in the pre-operative assessment of a potential transplant recipient?
- a Cytomegalovirus (CMV)
- b Hepatitis A
- c Hepatitis B
- d Hepatitis C
- e HIV

7 Which of the following are signs and symptoms of PVD?
- a Painless ulcers
- b Sunset foot
- c Buerger's angle <20 degrees
- d Clawed toes
- e Absent pulses

8 Which test may be helpful in the diagnosis of DVT?
- a Anti Xa activity
- b Platelet count
- c D-dimer
- d Prothrombin time
- e Activated partial thromboplastin time (APTT)

9 Which of the following regarding fat embolism is not true?
- a Commonly associated with long bone fractures
- b Causes haemorrhagic skin eruption
- c Causes fever
- d Commonly due to acute pancreatitis
- e Significant clinical consequences are rare

10 Which of the following are components of Well's score?
- a Pitting oedema greater in the symptomatic leg
- b Recent immobilisation for more than 3 days
- c Major surgery within 4 weeks
- d Calf swelling >3 cm compared to asymptomatic leg
- e Previous malignancy

Answers

SAQs

1 a Ruptured aortic aneurysm – most likely
Renal colic
Acute pancreatitis
Aortic dissection
Ruptured viscera
Perforated duodenal ulcer

b Male sex (4:1 male:female ratio)
Hypertension
PVD
Connective tissues disorders e.g. Marfan's syndrome
Family history
Age
Heart disease
Smoking

c Abdominal USS – a useful screening tool
CT scan/spiral CT scan
Focused assessment sonography in trauma (FAST scan) – may be
useful in acute rupture to identify free fluid in the abdomen
NB: Abdominal radiograph – may coincidentally identify an AAA
that is calcified, NOT used routinely in the formal assessment of an
AAA

d Marfan's syndrome

AAAs are thought to have a prevalence of around 5% in men aged 65 years. They are more common in men with male:female ratio of 4:1. By definition, an AAA is an increase in the aortic diameter by more than 150% of its original size. Risk factors include hypertension, PVD, family history, hyperlipidaemia, diabetes mellitus, smoking and connective tissue disorders such as Marfan's syndrome and Ehlers–Danlos syndrome. Common sites of aneurysms include aorta, iliac, popliteal and femoral. Most aneurysms are asymptomatic and are detected incidentally or due to complications such as thromboembolism or rupture. The UK Small Aneurysm Trial found that aneurysms < 5.5 cm diameter can be safely managed with regular examination and imaging. For aneurysms >5.5 cm risk of spontaneous rupture is greater and elective surgical repair is recommended. Other indications for surgery include rupture, symptomatic and rapidly expanding aneurysms. Endovascular repair of AAAs is now commonplace.

2 a Intermittent claudication
  b Hypertension
   Hypercholesterolaemia
   IHD
   Cerebrovascular disease
   Diabetes mellitus
   Systemic vasculitides
  c ABPI is the ratio of the blood pressure in the lower legs to the blood pressure in the arms.
   Lower blood pressure in the legs when compared to the arms is an indication of stenosed arteries secondary to PVD. It is calculated by dividing the systolic blood pressure at the ankle by the systolic blood pressures in the arm.
  d ABPI may be falsely elevated in diabetic patients due to arterial calcification.
  e Stop smoking
   Healthy balanced diet
   Weight loss
   Excellent diabetic control
   Increase exercise
   Walk through the pain to improve collateral circulation

PVD is commonly caused by atherosclerosis, occasionally fibromuscular dysplasia and vasculitides. Symptoms include cramping pains in the calves which usually comes on at a predictable distance; referred to as the claudication distance. Pain may also be felt in the buttocks and thighs. Ulceration, gangrene and rest pain are classical features of critical limb ischaemia. Signs of PVD include absent pulses; pallor; cold skin; atrophic skin; punched-out ulcers; Buerger's angle <20 degrees; and prolonged capillary refill time. Buerger's test involves raising the foot with the leg fully extended until the foot turns white, the foot is then slowly dropped. The angle at which colour returns to the foot is called the Buerger's angle. ABPI is a basic investigation that can be carried out to assess the severity of PVD. ABPI >1 = normal; 0.9–0.6 = claudication; 0.3–0.6 = rest pain and <0.3 = gangrene. Falsely elevated levels may occur due to arteriosclerosis as in diabetic patients.

3 a Embolus formation in the left atrium secondary to atrial fibrillation.
  b Pain
   Parasthaesia
   Perishingly cold
   Pallor
   Pulseless
   Paralysis

c IV heparin, 4–6 hourly APTTs
d Surgery – emergency embolectomy/endarterectomy/bypass graft
   Medical – intra-arterial tissue plasminogen activator
e Aspirin
   Statin
f Gas emboli
   Venous emboli
   Fat emboli
   Tumour emboli
   Amniotic fluid emboli

Acute limb ischaemia may be due to thrombosis, embolism or trauma. Signs and symptoms are summarised by the 'six Ps'. The presence of fixed mottling suggests irreversible limb ischaemia. Common sources of emboli include the heart secondary to AF and proximal aneurysms e.g. femoral, popliteal and aortic. Acute limb ischaemia is an emergency which requires urgent definitive management. If the diagnosis is in doubt request an urgent angiogram/arteriography. Embolic disease can be treated with surgical embolectomy or local tissue plasminogen activator. Thrombosis can be managed with urgent bypass or angioplasty depending on arterial run off. IV heparin should be commenced post-operatively. If embolic it is imperative to find the source – request echocardiography and an arterial duplex scan.

4 a Total Anterior Circulatory Syndrome
      b No – the bruit may be as a result of stenosis in the external carotid artery. A completed stenosed artery will also have no bruit as there is no flow.
      c To detect atrial fibrillation (AF) or heart block
         Pre-operative screen
      d LEFT carotid endarterectomy – patients should undergo carotid endarterectomy when they have a greater than 70% stenosis which is symptomatic. The patient's symptoms are right-sided, therefore, the embolus has come from the left carotid artery, hence a left carotid endarterectomy.
      e Smoking cessation
         Antihypertensives
         Lipid lowering agent
         Control diabetes
         Commence aspirin (stroke patients should receive 300 mg aspirin once daily for 2 weeks post-stroke)
         Treatment of AF with warfarin

Cerebral blood supply can be broadly divided into two parts; anterior circulation provided by the internal carotid arteries and posterior circulation provided by the basilar artery. Thrombus formation within the internal carotid arteries is a source of emboli which according to the site where emboli become lodged produce a variety of stroke syndromes summarised by the Oxford Classification of Stroke. The internal carotid artery has two terminal branches; anterior and middle cerebral arteries. Patients found to have carotid artery stenosis >70% should be referred to a vascular surgeon for consideration of carotid endarterectomy which significantly reduces the risk of stroke.

5 a Ulcers
Clawed foot
Poor/absent pulses
Sensory loss (especially vibration sense) in a stocking distribution
Absent ankle jerks
Loss of arches in feet
b Benzylpenicillin
Flucloxacillin
Metronidazole
Cefuroxime (or another IV cephalosporin) in penicillin sensitive individuals
c Maintain excellent glycaemic control
Inspect feet daily
Test bath water with hands instead of feet
Wear comfortable shoes with foot protection/cushioning soles
No barefoot walking
Regular chiropody to remove calluses and cut nails
Treat fungal infections early and aggressively
d Charcot's joint

Patients with diabetes mellitus are at risk of developing peripheral neuropathy and macro- and micro-vascular disease. To treat patients appropriately, it is vital to distinguish between ischaemia and peripheral neuropathy. Neuropathy is the result of vascular disease within the vasa nervorum (small arteries which supply peripheral nerves with blood) and chronic hyperglycaemia which leads to the increased formation of sorbitol and fructose in Schwann cells which disrupts nervous function. Signs and symptoms of diabetic foot disease therefore depend upon the aetiology. Ischaemia is associated with claudication, rest pain, rubor (sunset foot), trophic changes and painful ulceration on the heels and toes. Neuropathy is associated with parathesiae, pes cavus, clawed toes and painless ulceration typically over the bases of the metatarsals. Charcot's joint describes a neuropathic joint which has no nervous supply. The affected joint becomes destroyed due to increased range of movement and excessive mechanical stress, leading to severe joint deformity. Other causes of Charcot's joint include tabes dorsalis, syringomyelia and leprosy.

6 a Varicose eczema
Haemosiderin staining
Phlebitis
Atrophie blanche
Oedema
Varicose veins

b Short saphenous system – short saphenous vein runs posterior to lateral malleolus and ascends the posterior aspect of the calf to drain into the popliteal vein.

c Venous doppler USS – to assess presence of venous reflux, assess patency of femoral and popliteal veins and to assess status of perforating veins.
Venous duplex USS – allows the flow rate and anatomy to be accurately measured.

d Blood from superficial veins pass into deep veins via perforating veins. Valves within the walls of veins prevent retrograde blood flow from deep veins to superficial veins. However, if these valves become incompetent then this leads to venous hypertension and overdistension of superficial veins causing varicosities. Hypertension leads to oedema due to pressure within vessels exceeding interstitial pressure.

e Marjolin's ulcer – a squamous cell carcinoma arising at sites of chronic inflammation. Recognised causes include chronic venous disease, burns and osteomyelitis (OM).

The superficial venous drainage of the leg is via the long and short saphenous systems. A basic appreciation of the anatomy of these veins will enable you to identify which system is affected. The long saphenous vein begins on the medial aspect of the foot from the medial part of dorsal venous arch. It passes anterior to the medial malleolus accompanied by the saphenous nerve, a branch of the femoral nerve. It ascends the medial part of leg and thigh, passing about a hands breadth posterior to the patella. It terminates at the saphenofemoral junction. The short saphenous vein begins at the lateral part of the dorsal venous arch and ascends the leg posterior to the lateral malleolus. It terminates in the popliteal fossa where it drains into the popliteal vein. It is accompanied by the sural nerve, a branch of the tibial nerve. Varicosities will follow the path of the corresponding vein.

7 a   DVT
            Ruptured Baker's cyst
            Cellulitis
            NB: These conditions may co-exist
     b   D-dimer
            This would be elevated in any patient post-operatively.
     c   Stop the oral contraceptive pill 4 weeks prior to surgery and
            provide appropriate contraceptive advice.
            Early mobilisation post-operatively.
            Daily low molecular weight heparin (LMWH) as per local
            guidelines.
            TED stockings
            Adequate hydration
     d   Commence treatment dose LMWH/IV unfractionated heparin
            with warfarin simultaneously.
            Target international normalised ratio 2-3.
            Treat for 3 months post-operatively, 6 months if no cause can be
            found.

DVTs are more common in the post-operative period, where patients
must be assessed clinically for the condition. D-dimers, a commonly
used blood test to detect thromboembolic events are not accurate in
surgical patients as they will be falsely positive due to the necessity for
clot formation at the operation site.

8 a   Increasing age
            Pregnancy
            COCP/HRT use
            Surgery
            Previous DVT
            Malignancy
            Obesity
            Immobility
            Thrombophilias
     b   Well's score
     c   Calf warmth
            Calf tenderness
            Calf swelling
            Calf erythema
            Mild pyrexia
            Pitting oedema
     d   Pain on passive dorsiflexion of the foot on the affected side.
     e   Venous doppler ultrasound

DVT is a common surgical complication. Venous thrombosis formation depends upon the presence of Virchow's triad: venous stasis; hypercoagulable state and endothelial damage. Venous stasis is increased post-operatively due to immobility, and inflammatory mediators released post-operatively induce a hypercoagulable state. Venous thromboembolism (VTE) prophylaxis is a vital part of all patients care; all patients should be accurately assessed for the risk of VTE and an appropriate dose of LMWH should be prescribed and TED stockings given.

9 a Raynaud's syndrome
   b Systemic sclerosis
      SLE
      Thoracic outlet syndrome
      Sjogren's syndrome
   c Z-thumb
      Swan neck deformity
      Boutonniere deformity
      Ulnar deviation
      Splinter haemorrhages
      Rheumatoid nodules
   d Avoid triggers – e.g. cold, stress
      Stop smoking
      Wear gloves to keep hands warm
   e ESR
      Anti-nuclear antibodies
      Electrophoresis, cold agglutinins and fibrinogen may help identify a hyperviscosity state.
      Chest X-ray – cervical rib
   f Nifedipine
      Losartan
      Prazosin
      Fluoxetine
      Iloprost

Raynaud's syndrome describes peripheral digital ischaemia secondary to arterial spasm which may be precipitated by cold or stress. Patients report pain in their fingers and toes associated with colour changes. It may be primary/idiopathic or secondary and associated with connective tissue disorder such as systemic sclerosis, SLE, rheumatoid arthritis or other disorders such as thoracic outlet syndrome, Buerger's disease, thrombocytosis, or hypothyroidism. Management should include educating the patient about the avoidance of important triggers such as cold weather, and smoking cessation. In severe disease calcium channel blockers such as nifedipine may be useful in preventing arterial spasm. In refractory cases IV infusions of iloprost, a prostaglandin analogue which causes vasodilatation, can be used.

10 a Hypertension
Diabetes mellitus
Glomerulonephritis
   b Glomerular filtration rate < 15 ml/min
   c Virology status – HIV, hepatitis B and C, CMV
ABO blood group
HLA tissue typing
   d Tacrolimus
Cyclosporin
Azathioprine
Mycophenolate mofetil
Prednisolone
   e Opportunistic infection
Neoplasia/post-transplant lymphoproliferative disorder
Renal failure

Chronic renal failure is classified into five stages. End-stage renal failure is when renal replacement therapy is required for life and is defined as a glomerular filtration rate of <15 ml/min. Common causes include diabetes mellitus, glomerulonephritis, hypertension, renovascular disease, polycystic kidney disease and pyelonephritis. Rarer causes include myeloma, SLE, gout, vasculitis. Renal transplant is the treatment of choice for patients with end-stage renal disease. Contraindications to transplant include cancer, active kidney infection, severe heart disease or other co-morbidities. Donation is frequently from living related donors due to the small number of cadaveric kidneys available as a result of a small donor pool. Commonly used immunosuppressants include cyclosporin and tacrolimus, both calcineurin inhibitors which cause nephrotoxicity, and azathioprine, mycophenolate and prednisolone. There are many important short and long term complications which mean long term follow up is vital. Long-term complications include infection and malignancy and occur as a result of long-term immunosuppression.

EMQs

1	**A**	10	**C**	19	**F**
2	**E**	11	**B**	20	**G**
3	**F**	12	**I**	21	**G**
4	**D**	13	**C**	22	**E**
5	**C**	14	**C**	23	**C**
6	**A**	15	**B**	24	**A**
7	**B**	16	**A**	25	**H**
8	**E**	17	**C**		
9	**D**	18	**E**		

MCQs

1 e – Aneurysms can occur in any blood vessel, causing an increased risk of rupture. Saccular aneurysms are an outpouching of the blood vessel, most commonly found in Berry aneurysms. Fusiform aneurysms are a dilatation of the vessel. A dissecting aneurysm is where the arterial wall tears. A mycotic aneurysm is a localised dilatation due to destruction of the vessel wall by infection.

2 c – The risk factors for PVD include, smoking, age, diabetes, hypercholesterolaemia, hypertension, male, obesity, family history, stroke, and MI.

3 b – The branches of the abdominal aorta are the inferior phrenic arteries, coeliac trunk, superior mesenteric artery, suprarenal arteries, renal arteries, gonadal artery, inferior mesenteric artery, lumbar arteries, median sacral artery, and the common iliacs.

4 c – Noradrenaline is not a treatment for Raynaud's syndrome.

5 d – The signs of acute limb ischaemia are pain, pallor, perishingly cold, pulseless, paraesthesia, and paralysis, along with mottling of the limb.

6 a, c, d and e – It is essential that patients are thoroughly assessed prior to organ donation and organ transplantation to reduce the risk of rejection.

7 b, c and e – PVD typically presents with intermittent claudication, however, there may be arterial ulcers, discolouration of the limb, weak or absent distal pulses, loss of hair, or gangrene.

8 c – The D-dimer may be a useful test to indicate DVT. However, it is very non-specific, and may be raised due to inflammation or recent surgery.

9 d – Fat embolism is most commonly due to long bone fracture.

10 a, b, c and d – The Well's score is used for predicting the probability of having a DVT.

Chapter 5

Urology

Laura Dalton

SAQs

1 A 67-year-old man presents with urinary symptoms typically associated with benign prostatic hypertension (BPH).

   a Suggest three urinary symptoms that this patient may report. (3 marks)

   b Explain why urinary symptoms typically present earlier in BPH than in prostate carcinoma. (2 marks)

   c Suggest three useful investigations. (3 marks)

   d Give two methods of managing symptomatic BPH. (2 marks)

2 A 32-year-old man presents with a 3-day history of worsening left-sided testicular pain, dysuria and fever. On examination, he is pyrexial, with a swollen, warm and tender left testicle. A diagnosis of epididymo-orchitis is suspected.

   a List three alternative differential diagnoses for a swollen testicle. (3 marks)

   b Suggest two precipitating factors for epididymo-orchitis. (2 marks)

   c Suggest three investigations that may be useful. (3 marks)

   d Left untreated, epididymo-orchitis can lead to complications. List two. (2 marks)

3 A 67-year-old man presents with haematuria.

   a Name the two classifications of haematuria. (2 marks)

   b Suggest three differential diagnoses for haematuria. (3 marks)

   c What investigations would you request? Give three. (3 marks)

   d Name two complications of haematuria. (2 marks)

4 A 3-week-old boy presents with a left-sided scrotal swelling. On examination, the scrotum is fluctuant and can be transluminated. He does not appear to be in significant pain.

   a Explain the difference between a primary and secondary hydrocoele. (3 marks)

    b How can you distinguish between a hydrocoele and
        haematocoele clinically?   (1 mark)
    c List four differential diagnoses of scrotal swelling in any
        age group.   (4 marks)
    d Suggest two ways of managing a hydrocoele.   (2 marks)

5 A 71-year-old man presents with a history of urinary symptoms and back pain. Clinical examination reveals tenderness over the L4 and L5 vertebrae, and on rectal examination a large, hard, irregular prostate is palpable.
    a Suggest three investigations that you would request.   (3 marks)
    b A diagnosis of prostate carcinoma is made. Where does
        this typically metastasise to? Name two.   (2 marks)
    c Suggest an investigation used to stage the disease.   (1 mark)
    d Name the grading system used to stage prostatic
        carcinoma.   (1 mark)
    e Suggest three management options. These may be
        active or symptomatic.   (3 marks)

6 A 55-year-old woman presents with a history of haematuria, left-sided loin pain and unintentional weight loss over the last 3 months. Renal cell carcinoma is suspected.
    a Suggest two other differential diagnoses for someone
        presenting with haematuria.   (2 marks)
    b Suggest two bedside investigations.   (2 marks)
    c Suggest two useful radiological investigations for this
        patient.   (2 marks)
    d Suggest one medical and one surgical management
        option for renal cell carcinoma.   (2 marks)
    e Name two common sites for metastasis of renal cell
        carcinoma.   (2 marks)

7 A 43-year-old woman presents to A&E with a 2-day history of worsening right-sided flank and RUQ pain, with associated vomiting. On examination, she has right renal angle and right-sided abdominal pain.
    a Give four differential diagnoses for this patient other
        than renal colic.   (4 marks)
    b What three investigations will you request?   (3 marks)
    c Name three types of renal stone.   (3 marks)
    d Give two management options for renal calculi.   (2 marks)

8 A 15-year-old boy presents with sudden onset of right-sided testicular pain and swelling following playing a game of football. He is not sexually active and denies the presence of urinary symptoms. He is systemically well and apyrexial, but is in a significant amount of pain. On examination, the right testicle is swollen, firm and extremely tender.

    a Suggest two differential diagnoses other than testicular torsion. (2 marks)

    b Give three reasons suggested from the history and examination why torsion is most likely. (3 marks)

    c In the event of a suspected torsion, what is the gold standard investigation, and in what time frame should this be carried out? (2 marks)

    d Explain how torsion may lead to loss of the testicle. (3 marks)

9 A 58-year-old lady presents to her GP complaining of problems with urinary incontinence.

    a Suggest two further things you would ask in your history. (2 marks)

    b Explain how urinary continence and voiding is normally controlled. (4 marks)

    c Give four risk factors/causes of urinary incontinence. (2 marks)

    d Suggest two management options for urinary incontinence. (2 marks)

10 A 24-year-old man presents to his GP with a painless lump in his left testicle. A testicular tumour is suspected.

    a Give three other differential diagnoses of a testicular lump. (3 marks)

    b Name two types of testicular tumour. (2 marks)

    c Suggest two useful investigations for this patient. (2 marks)

    d Give three management options for testicular tumours. (3 marks)

    e Suggest two complications of a testicular malignancy or its treatments. (2 marks)

11 A 27-year-old girl is admitted with severe left flank pain, dysuria, and fever. She has complained of a stinging sensation when passing water for the past few days.

    a What is the most likely diagnosis? (1 mark)

    b Give three investigations you will request on admission to aid you with this diagnosis. (3 marks)

    c Name two common organisms causing this diagnosis. (2 marks)

    d List two possible complications of this condition. (2 marks)

    e Other than antibiotics give three important aspects of management for this condition. (3 marks)

12 A 34-year-old lady has been admitted with polycystic kidney disease. Her mother had the same condition.
   a Explain how this condition is inherited. (1 mark)
   b How may a patient present with polycystic kidney disease? (2 marks)
   c Give two ways in which you may diagnose this condition. (2 marks)
   d Give two aspects of your long-term management for this patient. Please give two long-term complications of this condition. (2 marks)
   e Cysts may occur in other locations in this condition. Please name one of these. (1 mark)

13 A 68-year-old lady comes to see you in the GP clinic complaining of a burning sensation when passing urine, which smells offensive. She is otherwise well, and denies haematuria.
   a What immediate investigation would you like to do? (1 mark)
   b Give three abnormalities you would expect to find on this investigation. (3 marks)
   c Name two common antibiotics used for this condition. (2 marks)
   d Please give three additional aspects of health advice you will give this lady. (3 marks)
   e In the paediatric population this diagnosis requires further investigation. Give three further things you would do in this circumstance. (3 marks)

EMQs

Select the most likely diagnosis for the following presentations:
A Haematocoele
B Testicular torsion
C Epididymo-orchitis
D Hydrocoele
E Testicular tumour
F Varicocoele

1 A 3-week-old boy develops a scrotal swelling. It appears to be painless and is transluminated when light is shone behind it.
2 A 16-year-old boy presents with sudden onset of pain in his left testicle. He denies being sexually active and has no symptoms of systemic infection.
3 A 21-year-old man presents with a painful lump in his right testicle. He reports having recent unprotected sexual intercourse and symptoms of dysuria and fevers.
4 A 29-year-old man finds a painless lump in his left testicle. He has no other symptoms.
5 A 43-year-old man complains of painful testicular swelling following trauma to the testis. It does not transluminate with light.

Select the most likely diagnosis for the following presentations:
A Renal stones
B Urinary tract trauma
C UTI
D Bladder carcinoma
E Renal cell carcinoma
F BPH

6 A 43-year-old woman presents with left-sided colicky flank pain and macroscopic haematuria.
7 A 17-year-old girl presents with a 3-day history of dysuria and frequency. Microscopic haematuria is found on urine dip.
8 A 73-year-old man presents with nocturia and macroscopic haematuria.
9 A 26-year-old man presents with macroscopic haematuria following an assault.
10 A 73-year-old ex-rubber manufacturer presents with painless frank haematuria.

Select the most likely diagnosis for the following presentations:
A Stress incontinence
B Urge incontinence
C Overactive bladder syndrome
D Functional incontinence
E Overflow incontinence
F True incontinence

11 A 93-year-old lady with severe osteoarthritis in both hips and dementia, who has recurrent episodes of irritability followed by incontinence.
12 A 33-year-old lady with a persistent leak of urine which is not controlled.
13 A 60-year-old man with frequent micturition due to a severe desire to urinate. He feels that when he has the sensation to void he must go immediately.
14 A 52-year-old lady who leaks small amounts of urine on sneezing and coughing.
15 A 65-year-old man with multiple sclerosis.

Select the most appropriate investigation for the following presentations:
A Ultrasound
B CT scan
C MRI
D Cystoscopy
E Surgical exploration
F Urine dip

16 A 17-year-old boy presents with a 2-hour history of severe sudden onset left testicular pain, with a retracted testicle.
17 A 26-year-old man with severe right loin to groin pain, with macroscopic haematuria.
18 An 18-year-old girl whose sister has just been diagnosed with polycystic kidney disease.
19 A 30-year-old lady with a first episode of dysuria and no other symptoms.
20 A 29-year-old man who presents with a painless lump in the left testicle.

Select the most likely diagnosis for the following presentations:
A Acute renal failure
B Chronic renal failure
C BPH
D Obstructing renal calculus
E Blocked catheter
F Renal cell carcinoma

21 You are called regarding a 72-year-old gentleman who is 2-days post op. He is well, although the nurse informs you that his urine output has been 0 ml over the past 3 hours, when it was previously 60 ml/hour.
22 A 68-year-old man who underwent an emergency repair of a suprarenal AAA yesterday. He has a low urine output and deteriorating renal function.
23 A 32-year-old girl with previously normal renal function, admitted with right loin to groin pain, microscopic haematuria, and a deteriorating renal function.
24 A 65-year-old man who has been unable to pass water for the past 24 hours. He presents with abdominal pain, and says he normally has nocturia and dribbling.
25 A patient admitted with frank haematuria, weight loss, and low Hb with a low MCV.

MCQs

1 What is the most useful first investigation you would do for a woman presenting with dysuria and frequency?
 a Urine dipstick
 b Bloods
 c Ultrasound KUB
 d Cystoscopy
 e CT scan

2 What investigation is most useful in staging carcinoma of the bladder?
 a CT scan
 b Ultrasound
 c Biopsy
 d Bone scan
 e MRI

3 What is the name of the staging system used in prostate carcinoma?
 a Dukes
 b TNM
 c Gleason
 d Ann Arbor
 e Breslow

4 What investigation is most appropriate when suspecting testicular torsion?
 a Ultrasound
 b Surgical exploration
 c Biopsy
 d CT scan
 e MRI

5 What is the most likely cause of a testicular swelling which transilluminates?
 a Haematocoele
 b Epididymo-orchitis
 c Hydrocoele
 d Testicular tumour
 e Scrotal hernia

6 What is the most common type of renal stone?
  a Cysteine
  b Calcium phosphate
  c Uric acid
  d Calcium oxalate
  e Struvite

7 What type of urinary incontinence is most likely with symptoms of leaking urine when coughing?
  a Urge incontinence
  b Stress incontinence
  c Mixed incontinence
  d True incontinence

8 Which is the most common type of testicular tumour?
  a Seminoma
  b Leydig
  c Sertoli cell
  d Sarcoma

9 In what time-frame should a suspected testicular torsion be explored before infarction is likely to occur?
  a 12 hours
  b 6 hours
  c 36 hours
  d 24 hours

10 Where does carcinoma of the prostate most commonly metastasise to?
  a Bone
  b Brain
  c Kidney
  d Lung

Answers

SAQs

1 **a** Nocturia
Frequency
Post-micturition dribbling
Hesitancy
Poor stream
Urinary retention

    b BPH usually affects the central zone of the prostate, meaning that the urethra becomes obstructed earlier, resulting in urinary symptoms presenting earlier.
Prostate carcinoma typically affects the peripheral zone of the gland and so occludes the urethra at a later stage.

    c FBC – raised white cells may make a UTI a possible explanation for the urinary symptoms
U+E – reduced renal function may be present because of obstructive uropathy and subsequent hydronephrosis and renal impairment
Urine dip and mid-stream urine (MSU) – evidence of infection may be present
Transrectal ultrasound (TRUS) scan guided biopsy of the prostate – histological evidence of malignancy
CT scan – useful in staging a possible prostate carcinoma

    d Transurethral resection of prostate (TURP)
Alpha-blocker such as Tamsulosin
5-alpha-reductase inhibitors such as Finasteride
Intermittent self-catheterisation
Long-term catheter

BPH is a common problem affecting men over the age of 60 years. Clinical features include frequency, nocturia, hesitancy, poor stream, post-void dribbling, acute retention and haematuria. The prostate usually feels enlarged but smooth on rectal examination. Management options include watchful waiting, alpha-blockers such as tamsulosin, 5-alpha–reductase inhibitors such as finasteride and TURP.

2 **a** Testicular torsion
Hydrocoele
Haematocoele

      Hernia
      Hydatid of Morgagni
      Varicocoele
      Epididymal cyst

b UTI
      Sexually transmitted infection (STI)
      Mumps infection
      Urethral obstructions leading to UTI
      After urethral procedures

c Urine dip and MSU – looking for evidence of infection and possible sensitivities
      Urethral swabs for STI
      USS of testes – looking for appearances of epididymo-orchitis, doppler to assess blood flow to testis
      Flexible cystoscopy – looking for urethral obstructions, which may have precipitated UTI

d Abscess
      Reduced fertility in affected scrotum, especially in the case of mumps infection.
      Chronic inflammation
      Necrosis

Epididymo-orchitis is inflammation of the epididymis and testis. It is commonly secondary to UTI. It may also develop following an STI or following prostatectomy. It is more common in those with urethral obstruction such as a stricture, or following urethral procedures.

It most frequently develops in association with an initial epididymitis which later spreads to the testis. In most cases, it resolves spontaneously or with antibiotics.

3 **a** Frank/macroscopic/visible haematuria
      Microscopic haematuria

   b Renal stones
      UTI
      Bladder carcinoma
      Renal cell carcinoma
      Urethral trauma/any trauma to renal tract
      Clotting abnormalities

   c Urine dip and MSU – the presence of white cells may indicate infection
      Urine cytology – evidence of malignant cells
      Ultrasound/CT scan – looking for renal stones, malignancy

    Cystoscopy – may show evidence of bladder tumours
    Ureteroscopy – may show ureteric or renal stones
d   Anaemia
    Clot retention
    Hypovolaemic shock

Haematuria is a common symptom, associated with a number of conditions affecting the urinary system. It may be visible (frank/macroscopic) or may only be detected on urine dip or microscopy (microscopic). Anaemia may result from large loss of blood via the urinary tract. Clots may cause obstruction of the urinary tract, resulting in urinary retention.

4 a   Primary – appears in the first few weeks of life, due to persistent processus vaginalis
           Secondary – due to underlying inflammation or neoplasm
       b   Hydrocoele can be transilluminated, haematocoele cannot
       c   Hernia
           Hydrocoele
           Haematocoele
           Varicocoele
           Epididymo-orchitis
           Epididymal cyst
           Torsion of hydatid of Morgagni
           Tumours of testis or spermatic cord
       d   Conservative – many newborn hydrocoeles resolve before 1 year of age
           Scrotal support
           Therapeutic aspiration
           Surgical removal of the hydrocoele by either a Jaboulay or Lord's procedure.
           Treat underlying cause i.e. give antibiotics if the underlying cause is infective.

A hydrocoele is an accumulation of serous fluid within the tunica vaginalis of the testis. Clinically, there is a smooth swelling which is usually fluctuant and can be transluminated.

   A primary hydrocoele appears in the first few weeks of life and results from the persistence of the processus vaginalis. A secondary hydrocoele can form at any age and may be associated with an underlying torsion, inflammation or malignancy.

   An acute inflammatory hydrocoele accumulates rapidly and may produce pain. A chronic hydrocoele causes gradual stretching of the tunica. It tends to cause a dragging sensation rather than pain.

5 a Urine dip and MSU – looking for evidence of infection and presence of haematuria
Prostate specific antigen – this is a marker of prostatic inflammation, but is not specific for malignancy
U+E – renal function may be impaired if there has been obstruction of the renal tract and high pressure retention
CT scan – useful in staging carcinoma
TRUS scan guided biopsy of the prostate – provides tissue for histological examination
Cystoscopy – may show enlargement of the prostate and local spread into the bladder and urethra
b Local spread to bladder, urethra, rectum
Lymph nodes
Distant metastasis to lungs, bone
c TRUS biopsy
CT scan
Bone scan
d Gleason grading
e Conservative – watchful waiting
LHRH analogues
Brachytherapy
Radical prostatectomy
TURP

By the age of 80 years, 80% of men have malignant foci within the prostate gland. This is typically an adenocarcinoma. Clinical features include those of urinary tract obstruction and of metastatic spread to bone. On rectal examination, the prostate feels hard and irregular.

Gleason grading stages the disease according to the cellular differentiation. A low score indicates a better prognosis.

Spread may be local to the urethra, bladder or seminal vesicle, lymphatic to sacral, iliac and para-aortic nodes, or distant, typically to bone, lungs and liver.

Management options include active surveillance, LHRH analogues in hormone-sensitive disease, radiotherapy or prostatectomy.

6 a UTI
Renal stones
Bladder carcinoma
Clotting abnormalities
Trauma
b Urine dip and MSU – looking for evidence of UTI
Urinary cytology – looking for evidence of malignant cells

FBC – raised white cell count may indicate infection, Anaemia may be present as a result of blood loss from haematuria, or as an effect of malignancy

U+E – deranged renal function may be present as a result of obstruction from malignancy or stones

LFT – if malignancy is present, deranged LFTs may indicate the possibility of liver metastases

c USS – may detect the presence of a mass, and can show the patency of the renal vein and inferior vena cava

IV urogram – will show the presence of a space-occupying lesion (SOL) within the kidney or ureter

CT/MRI – useful for staging malignant disease

d Medical – interleukin-2, β-interferon, tyrosine kinase

Surgical – radical/partial nephrectomy, percutaneous radiofrequency ablation

e Lymph nodes

Lungs

Liver

Bone

Brain

Renal cell carcinoma may present with haematuria, loin pain, a mass in the flank, malaise, anorexia and weight loss. Radiological investigations are helpful in identifying the site of the malignancy, assessing the patency of the renal vein and IVC and in staging the disease.

In local disease, nephrectomy is usually the preferred management option. A partial nephrectomy is advised if the contralateral renal function is poor. Interleukin-2 and β-interferon have been seen to cause remission in about 20% of cases.

The 5-year survival rate can be as high as 60–70% in tumours confined to the parenchyma. However, the rate is only 5% in those with metastatic disease.

7 a Cholecystitis/biliary colic

Pancreatitis

Appendicitis

Ovarian cyst

Ectopic pregnancy

b Urine dipstick and MSU – looking for signs of infection, blood may make a diagnosis of renal stones more likely

β-HCG – important to rule out pregnancy in women of reproductive age

Abdominal X-ray – may show radio-opaque stones, bowel obstruction, faecal loading

Ultrasound – may show presence of gallstones, ectopic pregnancy if β-HCG is positive, can identify hydronephrosis and renal calculi
CT KUB – will show the presence of renal stones and associated hydronephrosis, pancreatitis, appendicitis, ovarian cyst
Bloods – raised WCC may indicate infection, deranged LFTs makes a biliary source of symptoms more likely, raised amylase indicates pancreatitis

c   Calcium oxalate
    Urate
    Cysteine
    Calcium phosphate
d   Conservative – allow the stones to pass naturally
    Analgesia
    Antibiotic therapy – for UTI if present
    Ureteric stenting – reduce and prevent hydronephrosis
    Extracorporeal shockwave lithotripsy
    Ureteroscopy and laser defragmentation

Renal stones are a common occurrence, with an incidence of about 1 in 20 women and 3 in 20 men. They are found more commonly in those with a family history of stones, those with recurrent UTIs, and those with medical conditions causing raised levels of calcium, oxalate, urate and cysteine, but this is uncommon. In many cases, stones will be small enough to pass out of the body naturally. In some cases, stones may cause obstruction, resulting in hydronephrosis. If left untreated, this can cause renal impairment, and this is a reason for treatment to be initiated. This may be in the form of bypassing the obstruction using ureteric stenting, or by breaking up the stones, allowing them to be passed from the body.

8 a   Epididymo-orchitis
           Hydrocoele
           Torted hydatid of Morgagni
           Varicocoele
           Haematocoele
           Epididymal cyst
       b   Sudden onset – an infective cause would be likely to take a more gradual onset
           Following exertion – contraction of the cremaster muscle
           No urinary symptoms
           Systemically well/apyrexial
       c   Surgical exploration
           Within 6 hours from onset

   d Initial occlusion of the venous return
Rising pressure within the tunica
Impaired arterial supply
Necrosis of the tissues leading to shrunken fibrotic testis and
epididymis

Testicular torsion is an acute surgical emergency. It occurs typically in
adolescent boys aged 13–16, with an earlier peak at 1 year of age.

Predisposing factors include maldescent of the testis, an abnormally
long spermatic cord and an abnormally long mesorchium.

Initial occlusion of the venous return from the testis results in rising
pressure, causing impairment of the arterial supply.

If treatment is delayed the infarction progresses, resulting in
irreversible necrosis of the testis. Patients with suspected torsion should
undergo urgent surgical exploration and fixation of testis if torsion is in
fact present.

9 **a** Type of incontinence – differentiate between urge incontinence and
stress incontinence – does she find it difficult to get to the toilet on
time? Does she lose urine on laughing/coughing etc?
Quantify – does she have to change her clothes? Does she use pads?
If so how many a day?
Other symptoms – dysuria, incomplete voiding, post-micturition
dribbling, nocturia
Pregnancy history – number of deliveries, type of delivery, tears?

   b Bladder fills, detrusor stretches
Sympathetic fibres cause the internal urethral sphincter to remain
contracted, and the detrusor to remain relaxed.
Signals sent to the brain indicating a full bladder.
Parasympathetic fibres cause contraction of the detrusor muscle and
relaxation of the internal urethral sphincter.
Voluntary muscle in the external urethral sphincter contracts until
the person is in a 'socially appropriate' place to void.
At this point, the external urethral sphincter relaxes and voiding can
take place.

   c Female
Prostate surgery
Hysterectomy
Neurological disease – stroke, dementia, Parkinson's
Immobility
High body mass index (BMI)
Pelvic tumours/prostate enlargement
Vaginal deliveries – use of forceps, high birth weight
Stool impaction

d Lifestyle changes – reduce caffeine intake, modify high or low-fluid intake, lose weight if BMI >30.

Bladder training – pelvic floor muscle exercises, scheduled voiding intervals with stepped increases.

Medical therapy – oxybutynin for detrusor instability, intravaginal oestrogens for women who have post-menopausal vaginal atrophy causing overactive bladder, duloxetine in stress incontinence.

Surgical therapy – retropubic mid-urethral tape or rectal fascial sling in stress incontinence, sacral nerve stimulation or augmentation cystoplasty in detrusor overactivity.

Urinary incontinence is a common problem and can impact on physical, psychological and social well-being. It is defined as the involuntary leaking of urine, and has several types: Functional (inability to get to toilet in time due to immobility etc.), urge (sudden desire to urinate), stress (leaking during exertion, laughing, coughing, sneezing), mixed (both urgency and stress), overactive bladder syndrome, overflow incontinence, or true incontinence (due to a urethral–vaginal fistula).

Risk factors or causes include a high BMI, being female, hysterectomy, prostate surgery, pelvic tumours, enlarged prostate, traumatic vaginal deliveries, and neurological disease.

Management options include a variety of lifestyle changes, bladder training, medical therapies or surgery.

10 a Haematocoele
Hydrocoele
Lymphoma
Torsion
Epididymal cyst
Infection (tuberculosis (TB), syphilis, mumps, epididymo-orchitis)
Hernia
b Seminoma
Teratoma
Leydig cell
Sertoli cell
Sarcoma
c Ultrasound
Histological examination from inguinal orchidectomy.
Tumour markers
Alpha feto protein (not produced from seminomas).
β-HCG
LDH

d   Counselling and support groups
    Inguinal orchidectomy
    Radiotherapy (for seminomas)
    Chemotherapy (bleomycin, cisplatin and etoposide)
    Active surveillance
    Sperm storage
    Testicular prosthesis
e   Carcinoma of the other testicle
    Infertility/subfertility
    Toxicity from radiotherapy
    Metastases
    Complications from chemotherapy – bleomycin can cause lung
    fibrosis, cisplatin can cause nerve, hearing or renal damage.

Testicular malignancies are the most common malignancies found in men aged 20–30 years. Ninety-five percent of these are germ cell tumours (seminomas or teratomas), while 5% are non-germ cell tumours (Leydig, sertoli cell, sarcomas).

Risk factors include maldescent of the testis, Klinefelter's, family history, infertility, infantile hernia, taller height, low birth weight, low maternal or paternal age, breech presentation and multiparity.

Symptoms include a painless lump, pain, a dragging sensation, recent trauma, hydrocoele, and gynaecomastia from β-HCG production.

Seminomas most commonly metastasise to the para-aortic nodes which may cause back pain. Teratomas generally metastasise to liver, lung, bone and brain.

11 a   Pyelonephritis
    b   Bloods (FBC, U+E, CRP)
        Urine dip
        MSU
        Blood culture
        Observations
        β-HCG
    c   *E. coli* (80–85%)
        Staphylococcus saprophyticus (5–10%)
        Klebsiella
        Enterococcus
        Proteus
    d   Acute renal failure
        Renal scarring
        Sepsis

Perinephric abscess
Recurrence of pyelonephritis
e   Analgesia
IV fluid
Thromboprophylaxis
Monitoring urine output

Pyelonephritis typically stems from an untreated UTI. Patients typically present with loin pain, dysuria, and systemic symptoms such as fever, rigors, nausea and vomiting, however, they may become septic, hypotensive and shocked. Treatment should be initiated rapidly to prevent deterioration of renal function by giving IV fluids, and treating the infection with IV antibiotics.

12 a   Autosomal dominant
b   Abdominal pain
Flank pain which may be bilateral
Nocturia
Haematuria
Drowsiness
Joint pain
Screening due to family history
c   Ultrasound
CT
MRI
Intravenous pyelogram
d   Antihypertensives
Diuretics
Low-salt diet
Prompt treatment of UTIs
Consider for renal transplant
e   Hypertension
Recurrent kidney infections
Chronic renal failure
Anaemia
Liver failure
f   Liver
Pancreas
Testes

Polycystic kidney disease is usually autosomal dominant, and often presents due to a positive family history, however, patients may be admitted with flank or abdominal pain, haematuria, or in renal failure.

Cysts can also form on the liver, pancreas and testes, causing their own complications.

13 a Urine dip
   b Leukocytes
     Nitrites
     Blood
     Protein
   c Trimethoprim
     Nitrofurantoin
     Amoxicillin
   d Wipe from front to back
     Wear cotton undergarments
     Urinate after intercourse
     Keep the genital area clean
     Drink plenty of fluids
     Drink cranberry juice
   e Referral to urologist
     Ultrasound of the kidneys
     Voiding cystourethrogram

UTIs are very common, usually due to spread from the GIT. They are more common in women due to the shorter urethra. There are several underlying predisposing factors which should be investigated in patients with recurrent episodes. These include diabetes, analgesic nephropathy, immunodeficiency, renal calculi, urinary obstruction, vesicoureteric reflux, pelvic ureteric junction obstruction, catheterisation, incomplete voiding, urinary stasis, and pregnancy.

EMQs

1	**D**	10	**D**	19	**F**
2	**B**	11	**D**	20	**A**
3	**C**	12	**F**	21	**E**
4	**E**	13	**B**	22	**A**
5	**A**	14	**A**	23	**D**
6	**A**	15	**E**	24	**C**
7	**C**	16	**E**	25	**F**
8	**F**	17	**B**		
9	**B**	18	**A**		

MCQs

1   a – Dysuria and frequency most commonly occur with a UTI, which may be easily detected on urine dipstick tests.

2   a – Bladder cancer staging is done by looking at the layers of the bladder involved, which is best identified on CT scan.

3   c – Dukes staging is for colorectal tumours, TNM is a generic staging tool, Ann Arbor staging is for lymphoma, Breslow thickness is for malignant melanomas.

4   b – Testicular torsion is a surgical emergency, with operative intervention the primary investigation, preferably performed within the first 6 hours of the onset of pain.

5   c – A hydrocele typically transilluminates brilliantly, and feels like a smooth uniform enlargement around the testicle.

6   d – Calcium oxalate stones account for almost 80% of renal calculi.

7   b – Stress incontinence is the most common form of incontinence, which typically occurs due to a sudden rise in intra-abdominal pressure, such as coughing or sneezing. The main treatment is to strengthen the pelvic floor muscles.

8   a – Seminoma is the most common testicular malignancy, typically occurring around the age of 40.

9   b – testicular torsion is a surgical emergency, with the blood supply requiring restoration within 6 hours of the onset of pain.

10   a – Prostate cancer typically metastasises to the bony pelvis and spine.

Chapter 6

Trauma and orthopaedic surgery

Nicholas Eastley

SAQs

1 Mavis, an 83-year-old lady with a previous wrist fracture, presented to the emergency department after falling over in her garden. She was found on the floor by her husband, and was unable to weight bear. An X-ray is performed which shows Mavis has an intracapsular fracture of her right hip.

    a   What other simple investigations would you perform in the emergency department? (3 marks)

    b   Name three painkillers which could be given to Mavis in the emergency department. (3 marks)

    c   What two risk factors does Mavis have for fracturing her hip? (2 marks)

    d   What is the blood supply to the femoral head? (3 marks)

    e   If the blood supply to the head of the femur is compromised, what late complication will occur? (1 mark)

    f   Name one operation suitable for the treatment of an intracapsular hip fracture. (1 mark)

    g   Post-operatively the on-call doctor is called to see Mavis as the nurses are concerned that she has become breathless and light headed. Her HR is 110, BP 100/60, RR 22 and Sats 92% on 6l O_2. She is clearly breathless and complaining of chest pain. Name three post-operative complications fitting with Mavis' symptoms. (3 marks)

    h   Physiotherapy is instigated on the first day post-operatively. Give three reasons this is so important. (3 marks)

2 Mike, a 34-year-old motorcyclist, has been brought to the emergency department after being knocked off his bike whilst travelling at 60 mph. On arrival, his GCS is 15 and he is complaining of pain in his groin. He subsequently has a pelvic X-ray which shows an intertrochanteric fracture of his left hip.

  a Give three signs suggesting a fractured neck of femur on clinical examination. (3 marks)

  b In general is the blood supply to the femoral head compromised in an intertrochanteric fracture? (1 mark)

  c What operation is most suitable to treat this kind of fracture? (1 mark)

  d Name four complications of this surgery that should be put on the consent form. (4 marks)

  e Three days post-operatively Mike starts to complain of increasing pain in his wound. On examination the skin surrounding the incision has become erythematous, and is warm to touch. Name three types of bacteria which can cause post-operative wound infections. (3 marks)

  f Name four common causes of post-operative pyrexia. (4 marks)

  g Name two suitable antibiotics which could be started to treat a superficial wound infection. (2 marks)

3 Edith, an obese 65-year-old lady, has fallen over outside her house while she was having a cigarette. She can't remember why she fell, but is complaining of a painful left wrist.

  a Name three fractures that occur after a fall onto an outstretched arm. (3 marks)

  b Name three signs which would suggest that Edith has fractured her wrist. (3 marks)

  c Edith has an X-ray of her wrist which has shown a fracture. The orthopaedic registrar on call diagnoses a Colles' fracture. What is the definition of a Colles' fracture? (2 marks)

  d Name four investigations which you would perform in the emergency department? (4 marks)

  e Edith is admitted and undergoes surgery to reduce and immobilise the fracture. The following night she starts to complain of 'pins and needles' in her left hand. She denies any pain but, on examination, her index finger is numb to light touch. Motor function and power is normal in the fingers. Describe what is causing this sensation disturbance. (2 marks)

  f What two conservative measures should be done to try and resolve the problem? (2 marks) g   Prior to discharge Edith is diagnosed as having osteoporosis. Other than the distal radius, name two bony areas which are classically affected by osteoporosis?   (2 marks)

h   Name two medications that reduce the effects of osteoporosis?   (2 marks)

i   Name three other conservative measures which will reduce the risk of Edith suffering further fractures caused by falls in the future?   (3 marks)

4   Jamie has come to the emergency department after falling from a swing. He is complaining of a painful left shin, and when you cut his trouser off you find a 4 cm bleeding wound midway between his knee and his ankle. X-rays confirm that he has an open fracture of his tibia and fibula at the junction of the middle and distal third of his lower limb. On examination, neurovascular status in his left foot is intact.

a   What classification system is used to describe open fractures?   (1 mark)

b   Give two additional areas of management you would need to include when managing an open fracture, compared with a closed injury.   (2 marks)

Jamie is admitted and undergoes emergency surgery. His wound is thoroughly cleaned and debrided, and the fractures internally reduced and fixed. The operating surgeon feels there is enough tissue to close the wound in theatre. His foot is documented as being 'neurovascularly intact' in recovery. The following night, you are on call and asked to see him after he starts to complain of very severe pain in his left lower leg and foot. On examination, his foot is cold and pale compared with the right. You are unable to locate any pulses in his foot with a Doppler.

a   Name the two pulses you would attempt to find in the foot on Doppler.   (2 marks)

b   What complication has most likely occurred?   (1 mark)

c   Name three areas in which this complication can occur.   (3 marks)

d   The registrar-on-call reviews the patient and decides surgical intervention is required. What operation needs to be performed immediately?   (2 marks)

5 Mary has come to see you in outpatients. She is complaining of an aching pain in her right hand that regularly wakes her up at night. She has also started to drop things at work, and states that she gets pins and needles in her fingers intermittently. On examination, there are findings consistent with carpal tunnel syndrome (CTS).

a   What nerve is encroached in CTS, and what is its motor
    and sensory distribution?   (5 marks)

b   List the contents of the carpal tunnel.   (5 marks)

c   Give five causes of CTS.   (5 marks)

d   Give two specific clinical tests used to help diagnose
    CTS.   (2 marks)

e   Name one other investigation that can be used to
    confirm the diagnosis of CTS.   (1mark)

f   Give three ways to treat CTS.   (3 marks)

6 Frank has come to clinic after being referred by his GP. Over the last 5 years he has developed bilateral knee pain. He is severely limited in his daily activities because of this pain. You order some X-rays of Frank's knees which show changes consistent with osteoarthritis.

a   Name three changes characteristically seen on an X-ray
    which suggest osteoarthritis?   (3 marks)

b   Name three types of analgaesia suitable for this patient.   (3 marks)

c   Give two ways that patients can improve the way the
    symptoms of osteoarthritis affect them.   (2 marks)

d   Give three joints commonly affected by osteoarthritis
    other than knees.   (3 marks)

7 Brian, aged 70, has attended his GP complaining of lower back pain. He is now particularly concerned as he has some numbness in his buttocks. When taking a history, you find that he has some long-standing urinary symptoms including hesitancy, poor stream and dribbling. He also complains of some recent weight loss. On examination, he has some reduced sensation to light touch over his perineum, although motor function is normal in his legs. When you see him you are concerned he may have cauda equina syndrome.

a   Name four red flags associated with cauda equina
    syndrome.   (4 marks)

b   What is the definition of a myotome and a dermatome?   (2 marks)

c   What is the myotome and dermatome of S1?   (2 marks)

d   Name three causes of cauda equina syndrome.   (3 marks)

e   Name one radiological investigation critical to
    investigate Brian's neurological symptoms further.   (1 mark)

8 You are called to the emergency department as part of the trauma team to help see John, a 30-year-old man, who has been involved in a car accident. On arrival, he has an obvious head injury and a deformed left ankle. His HR is 120, BP 90/60, Sats 90% on 10L of O_2 via a non re-breather mask, RR 24 Temp 36.7°C. His eyes only open when you apply supra-orbital pressure, at which point he also makes incomprehensible sounds, and tries to grab your hand. He is maintaining his own airway. The paramedics have applied a C-spine collar and blocks, and a pelvic binder at the scene of the accident.

a What is John's GCS? (1 mark)

When examining John you notice there is reduced movement of the right hand side of his chest on inspiration. He flinches when you palpate over the area, and on auscultation, there is reduced air entry on the right compared to the left. The right side of the chest is also dull to percussion.

b What pathology is most likely considering these findings and John's observations? (1 mark)

c What would you do to manage this? (1 mark)

d Give four X-rays you would request when John's condition stabilises. (4 marks)

e Suddenly John's GCS deteriorates and his airway becomes compromised. His HR falls to 40 BPM and BP increases to 160/80. Give four signs suggesting a patient has developed an obstructed airway. (4 marks)

f Name three ways you can attempt to maintain a compromised airway. (3 marks)

g After stabilisation, John has a CT scan of his head. A large cerebral haemorrhage is noted. What syndrome appears to have has occurred? (1 mark)

9 Lucinda has fallen off her horse and twisted her left ankle. She has hobbled into the emergency department where you use the Ottowa's rules to decide whether to do an X-ray.

a What are the indicators of performing an ankle X-ray according to the Ottowa's rules? (3 marks)

b You perform an X-ray and diagnose a fracture of Lucinda's left ankle. Name one classification system of ankle fractures. (1 mark)

c Name three of the ligaments which provide stability to the ankle joint. (3 marks)

d   The consultant-on-call decides that the fracture is
    unstable and needs open reduction and internal fixation.
    Two days post-operatively, she starts to complain of
    pain in her right calf. You are concerned she has a DVT.
    What investigation would you like to request to confirm
    this diagnosis?   (1 mark)

e   If confirmed, how would you immediately treat a DVT
    in the lower leg?   (1 mark)

10 Joan has come to see you in clinic after her GP referred her. She is
    complaining of pain in her fingers and, as a result, is now finding it difficult
    to use a knife and fork or her telephone. On further questioning, you find
    that the pain is worse in the mornings, affects both hands equally, and
    that Joan's fingers are often stiff and swollen. On examination, Joan has
    swollen proximal interphalangeal (PIP) and metacarpophalangeal (MCP)
    joints. You suspect rheumatoid arthritis.

a   Give three blood tests you would request and explain
    why.   (3 marks)

b   X-rays are carried out. Give three changes you would
    expect to find in rheumatoid arthritis.   (3 marks)

c   Give four extra-articular signs of rheumatoid arthritis.   (4 marks)

d   Give four conservative measures or treatments that
    would help Joan deal with rheumatoid arthritis.   (4 marks)

11 Fiona has fallen off her horse and is unable to move her right arm. Staff
    in the emergency department are concerned that she may have dislocated
    her glenohumeral joint.

a   What nerve is characteristically at risk of damage when
    a shoulder is dislocated?   (2 marks)

b   What area of skin is supplied by this nerve?   (1 mark)

c   Describe the two most common types of glenohumeral
    dislocation, including the mechanisms that classically
    cause each.   (4 marks)

Following X-rays, Fiona is diagnosed as having a dislocation of her
shoulder. There were no fractures visible. You decide to relocate the
shoulder in the emergency department.

d   Give two drugs that could be used to help facilitate the
    relocation.   (2 marks)

e   After the shoulder is relocated Fiona complains of a new
    pain in her left wrist. Another X-ray is performed, which
    shows a distal radius fracture, with anterior (palmar)
    displacement of the distal fragment. What is the name
    of this fracture?   (2 marks)

12 You are asked to see a medical inpatient, Sandra, who complains that for the last few years she has found it hard to completely extend the fingers on her right hand. On examination, you find thickened digital and palmar fascia on the hand. You also notice contractures and fixed deformities at the MCP and PIP joints of the middle and ring finger.

a   What disease does Sandra have? (1 mark)
b   Give five risk factors associated with this disease. (5 marks)
c   Which finger is most commonly affected? (1 mark)
d   Give one conservative treatment for the condition. (1 mark)
e   Give two surgical procedures that can used to treat this condition. (2 marks)

13 Louis, an amateur golfer, attends the emergency department complaining of pain in his left knee. The pain began whilst he was looking for his ball in the bushes at his local golf course. He denies any trauma whatsoever. He also complains of general malaise and feeling feverish. On examination, Louis' knee is warm to touch and very swollen. He is unable to flex his knee because of severe pain. His observations are HR 110, BP 140/80, RR 16, Sats 98% on air and temperature 39°C.

a   What is the most likely diagnosis? (1 mark)
b   Name two causative organisms of this condition. (2 marks)
c   Name five investigations you would immediately perform in the emergency department. (5 marks)
d   Name two suitable antibiotics which could be started. (2 marks)
e   Give two other differential diagnoses for a hot swollen warm knee joint. (2 marks)

14 Amy, aged 21, is a type one diabetic who has been brought in to the emergency department with a temperature of 38.5°C. She is a known intravenous drug user (IVDU) who admits injecting drugs into the veins in her legs. On examination, her chest sounds clear, and her urine dip is negative. She denies any diarrhoea or abdominal pain. On her thigh you notice a large erythematous swelling. The swelling is approximately 10 cm × 15 cm in size, and is tense, warm and tender on palpation. You diagnose this swelling as an abscess.

a   What is the management of abscesses in general? (1 mark)
b   What risk factors does Amy have for the development of complicated, recurrent abscesses? (2 marks)

Amy is operated on and admitted. Ten days post-operatively she remains pyrexial so you decide to perform an X-ray of the abscess cavity. The radiologist-on-call bleeps you to let you know they are concerned Amy has developed OM.

c   Give two signs you may see on a plain X-ray suggesting
     OM.   (2 marks)
d   List three bacteria that commonly cause acute OM.   (3 marks)
e   Outline five aspects of the management of acute OM.   (5 marks)

15 James has fallen whilst playing rugby and attended the emergency
department. After examining him you are concerned he has fractured his
scaphoid.
a   What clinical signs would you expect following a
     fractured scaphoid?   (3 marks)
b   A scaphoid series of X-rays are carried out and confirm a
     fracture. Describe the X-rays which make up a scaphoid
     series.   (4 marks)
c   Describe the blood supply of the scaphoid.   (1 mark)
d   Name two bones other than the scaphoid at risk of
     avascular necrosis.   (2 marks)
e   Name two early and two late complications of open
     reduction internal fixation of the scaphoid bone.   (4 marks)

EMQs

Match the appropriate GCS score with the clinical responses:
A   13
B   5
C   8
D   7
E   6
F   10
G   11
H   15

1   Eyes open spontaneously, localised pain, confused conversation.
2   Eyes open spontaneously, follows commands, orientated conversation.
3   Eyes open to pain, extensor response and inappropriate words to pain.
4   Eyes open to voice, normal flexor response to pain, confused conversation.
5   Eyes open and abnormal flexion to pain, no verbal response whatsoever.

Match the neurological deficits with the peripheral nerve injuries:
A Ulnar nerve damage at the elbow
B Radial nerve damage in the radial groove
C Axillary nerve compression in the axilla
D Median nerve damage in the wrist
E Musculocutaneous nerve damage in the axilla
F Anterior interosseous nerve damage
G Evulsion of lower roots of brachial plexus
H Evulsion of upper roots of brachial plexus

6 Reduced flexion and supination of the elbow. Reduced sensation over lateral forearm.
7 Deltoid paralysis and reduced sensation over the 'regimental badge' region.
8 Weakness of brachioradialis, supinator and all of the forearm extensors. Sensory disturbance on back of hand.
9 The formation of a characteristic 'claw hand' deformity.
10 Loss of sensation over the lateral three and a half digits, and inability to perform thumb opposition.

Match the motor supply to the nerve of the lower limb:
A Deep fibular (peroneal) nerve
B Femoral nerve
C Sciatic nerve
D Obturator nerve
E Superficial fibular (peroneal) nerve
F Tibial nerve
G Musculocutaneous nerve
H Superior gluteal nerve

11 Tibialis anterior.
12 Peroneus brevis.
13 Adductor longus.
14 Vastus lateralis.
15 Tensor fascia lata.

Match each spinal nerve with the area of skin it supplies sensation to:
A T12
B L4
C L5
D L3
E S5
F T10

G S1
H L1

16 Medial aspect lower limb.
17 Lateral aspect lower limb.
18 Anterior aspect of knee.
19 Umbilicus.
20 Symphysis pubis.

Match each muscle movement with the relevant spinal nerve:
A C5
B C6
C C7
D C8
E T1
F L2
G L3,4
H L5

21 Arm abduction.
22 Hip flexion.
23 Knee extension.
24 Ankle and big toe dorsiflexion.
25 Elbow extension.

MCQs

1 What classification system is used to classify scaphoid fractures?
  a Herbert's
  b Lauge Hansen
  c Weber's
  d Garden's
  e Neer's

2 You are concerned that a patient you are seeing in the emergency department has ruptured their Achilles tendon. What clinical test can you perform to confirm your diagnosis?
  a Lachman
  b McMurray
  c Thomson
  d Trendelenberg
  e Thomsen

3 Fractures involving the growth plate (the epiphyseal plate) in children can be classified using the Salter Harris system. How is a fracture which results in the displacement of the epiphyseal plate and part of the metaphyses grouped?

a   Salter Harris I
b   Salter Harris II
c   Salter Harris III
d   Salter Harris IV
e   Salter Harris V

4 A patient has attended the emergency department after accidentally lacerating his forearm whilst cutting wood. He complains he cannot 'cock his wrist backwards.' On examination, he cannot extend his wrist. What nerve has been damaged?

a   Ulnar
b   Radial
c   Median
d   Musculocutaneous
e   Anterior interosseous nerve

5 Which of the following is false regarding meniscal injuries in patients?

a   More common in men than women.
b   Usually results from a weight-bearing injury causing the patient to stop immediately.
c   The absence of knee swelling does not exclude meniscal tears.
d   Joint line tenderness is nearly always present.
e   A locked knee caused by meniscal injury should be treated conservatively with pressure supports and crutches.

6 A patient is brought to the emergency department after falling off his mountain bike. When you apply a painful stimulus his eyes do not open. He also moans and forms an abnormal flexor response. What is his GCS?

a   9
b   7
c   5
d   8
e   6

7 You are asked to reduce a dislocated shoulder in the emergency department. You use the technique you are most familiar with. You give suitable analgesia and then apply longitudinal traction and external rotation to the arm for several minutes. At 90° of external rotation, you adduct the arm whilst internally rotating the limb, at which point relocation occurs. What technique have you used?

   a   Stimson's

   b   Hippocratic

   c   Milch's

   d   Kocher's

   e   Bigelow's

8 Which of the following options accurately describes the normal range of movement of the hip joint?

   a   Flexion 120°, Extension 5-20°, Abduction 40°, Adduction 25°, Internal/External rotation at 90° flexion = 45°

   b   Flexion 100°, Extension 5-15°, Abduction 45°, Adduction 20°, Internal/External rotation at 90° flexion = 45°

   c   Flexion 110°, Extension 5-15°, Abduction 40°, Adduction 15°, Internal/External rotation at 90° flexion = 45°

   d   Flexion 120°, Extension 5-10°, Abduction 50°, Adduction 25°, Internal/External rotation at 90° flexion = 50°

   e   Flexion 120°, extension 5-20°, Abduction 30°, Adduction 30°, Internal/External rotation at 90° flexion = 45°

9 Non-union is a significant risk of fracture involving:

   a   Clavicle

   b   Distal radius

   c   Tibia

   d   Talus

   e   4th Metacarpal

10 Which of the following is true regarding congenital dislocation of the hip?

   a   Treatment is conservative with splinting applied after hip reduction

   b   Surgery should be performed immediately after the diagnosis is made

   c   The affected leg may appear longer than the unaffected side

   d   Trendelenberg's test is negative in older patients

   e   Ortolani and Patrick's tests are used for diagnosis

Answers

SAQs

1 **a** Bloods (FBC, U+Es, clotting, group and save)
       Chest X-ray
       ECG
   b Paracetamol
       NSAIDs
       Codeine phosphate
       Tramadol
       Oramorph
       Morphine sulphate
       Nitrous oxide
   c Age
       Sex
       Osteoporosis
   d Ligamentum teres vessels
       Medial circumflex artery
       Nutrient vessels
   e Avascular necrosis or the femoral head/osteoarthritis.
   f Hemiarthroplasty
       Total hip replacement
   g Acute coronary syndrome
       Aspiration pneumonia/lower respiratory tract infection (LRTI)
       Pulmonary embolism (PE)
   h Reduce risks of bed sores
       Reduces muscle wastage
       Prevents stiffness
       Reduces the risk of VTE disease
       Reduces the risk of pneumonia

Increasing age, worsening cognitive impairment and a reduced bone mass mean fractured neck of femurs are relatively common in the elderly. Approximately 15–20% of patients die within one year of a major fracture. Patient may also have permanent disability resulting from persistent pain and limited physical mobility. Patients who fracture their hip usually have co-existing medical comorbidities which mean they are often at higher risk of anaesthetic complications. Prophylactic LMWH, thromboembolic deterrent stockings and early mobilisation should be emphasised to the patient.

2   a   Inability to straight leg raise
          Shortened leg
          Externally rotated leg
          Groin tenderness
          Greater trochanter tenderness
   b   No
   c   The insertion of a Dynamic Hip Screw
   d   Pulmonary embolus
          DVT
          Infection
          Bleeding
          Scar
          Pain
          Mal-union
   e   *Staphylococcus aureus* (inc. MRSA)
          Pseudomonas aeruginosa
          Coagulase negative *staphylococcus*
          Streptococcus pyogenes
          Enterococci including *E. coli*
   f   UTI
          DVT
          Pneumonia/LRTI/atelectasis
          Cellulitis (surrounding cannula sites or surgical incisions)
   g   Flucloxacillin
          Benzylpenicillin
          Erythromycin

Superficial wound infection is a common cause of fever post-operatively. Deeper infections involving metalwork are a serious complication due to the absence of an adequate vasculature to supply antibiotics to the tissues involved. As a result, prophylactic antibiotics are often used when implanting metalwork or vascular grafts.

3   a   Scaphoid
          Distal radius
          Radial head
          Supracondylar region of humerus
          Neck of humerus
          Clavicular
   b   Swelling
          Erythema
          Tenderness
          Deformity (i.e. 'dinner fork' deformity in a Colles' fracture)

c A fracture of the distal radius, with dorsal (posterior) displacement and angulation of the distal fragment.

d Urine dip
Bloods – FBC/U+Es/CRP/group and save (Max 2 marks)
Chest X-ray
ECG

e Local swelling or excessively tight cast causing compression of the median nerve.

f Elevate the limb involved.
Split or remove any plaster cast or tight dressings.

g Neck of femur
Lumbar spine

h Bisphosphonates
Vitamin D supplements
Calcium supplements

i Physiotherapy to improve muscular strength and balance.
Occupational therapy involvement to address any risks for future falls i.e. suitable footwear, stairs.
Hip protectors
Lose weight
Healthy diet
Stop smoking

If the distal segment of the radius is stable, and its anatomical position is adequate, a Colles' fracture can be treated conservatively. Adequate analgaesia (often in the form of a Biers block) is given, and after closed reduction a plaster cast applied. If operative treatment is suitable, K-wires, plates and screws, or rarely an external fixator can be used. The neurovascular status of all limbs must be checked when a fracture has occurred, especially prior to and after any reduction.

4 a Gustillo's classification

b Give IV antibiotics
Wash out wound with copious amounts of sterile water or saline.
Photograph and then cover injury.

c Dorsalis pedis
Posterior tibial

d Compartment syndrome

e Abdomen
Lower limb
Forearm
Luteal
Thigh

f Open fasciotomy

Both open fractures and compartment syndrome are orthopaedic emergencies. An open fracture is a fracture that has a communication through the overlying skin with the environment. Compartment syndrome is elevation of interstitial pressure in a closed fascial compartment that results in microvascular compromise. Patients who are at high risk of compartment syndrome include those with circumferential burn injuries, high-energy lower limb fractures, crush injuries, and those with a reperfusion injury.

5   a   Median nerve
      Sensory – radial/lateral three and a half fingers
      Motor – pronator teres, pronator quadratus, all the flexor muscles in the forearm except flexor carpi radialis and the medial half of flexor digitorum
      Profundus
   b   Flexor carpi radialis
      Flexor pollicis longus
      Median nerve
      Flexor digitorum superficialis
      Flexor digitorum profundus
   c   Idiopathic
      Trauma
      Rheumatoid arthritis
      Acromegaly
      Myxoedema
      Diabetes mellitus
      Hypothyroidism
      Pregnancy
   d   Tinnel's and Phalen's tests
   e   Nerve conduction studies
   f   Corticosteroid injection
      Splint use
      Carpal tunnel decompression

The carpal bones form an arch in the wrist which is covered by a sheath of tough connective tissue called the flexor retinaculum. Wrist splints can be worn to keep the wrist straight, and subsequently reduce pressure on the median nerve as it passes through the tunnel. They can be worn either just at night or all day.

6 a Reduced joint space
        Subchondral bone sclerosis
        Cyst formation
        Osteophyte formation
     b Paracetamol
        Codeine phosphate
        Tramadol
        NSAIDs
     c Physiotherapy to strengthen muscles.
        Walking aids
        Stair lifts
        Heat therapy
        Losing weight
     d The lumbar spine
        The hip
        The first carpometacarpal joint

Osteoarthritis is defined as a chronic irreversible degenerative disease of articular cartilage. Predisposing factors include obesity, excessive heavy joint use, trauma, inflammatory arthritis, osteonecrosis, injection of intra-articular steroids, hyperparathyroidism and inheritable disorders of connective tissue. Pain on weight bearing is the classical symptom that patients complain of.

7 a Saddle anaesthesia
        Sphincter dysfunction including urinary retention, and faecal or urinary incontinence.
        Bilateral sciatica
        Motor weakness in the lower limbs.
        Loss of anal tone.
     b Myotome – each muscle in the body is supplied by a segment of the spinal cord and its corresponding spinal nerve. The muscle and this nerve make up a myotome.
        Dermatome – a dermatome is an area of skin that is mainly supplied by a single nerve root.
     c Myotome – plantar flexion of the foot
        Dermatome – the posterior calf and sole of foot
     d Infection and subsequent abscess formation
        Tumours
        Iatrogenic (lumbar puncture haematoma)
        Chronic inflammatory conditions of the spine, such as Paget's disease, ankylosing spondylitis, and spondylolisthesis.
        Disk herniation
     e MRI

Within the vertebral column, the spinal cord is transmitted in the spinal canal. Below the spinal cord, the spinal nerves slope inferiorly to their appropriate intervertebral foramina. At this point, they are known as the cauda equina. Urinary retention is the most consistent finding for cauda equina syndrome, although in any potential cauda equina syndrome it is important to examine for saddle anaesthesia, rectal tone, plus any of the other red flag symptoms.

8 a 9
   b Haemothorax
   c Insert a chest drain
   d Pelvis
      Chest
      Left ankle (AP and lateral)
      Cervical spine (AP and lateral)
   e Agitation secondary to hypoxia
      Tachypnoea
      Desaturations
      Cyanosis
      Gurgling (usually caused by secretions, vomit or blood)
      Stridor
      Respiratory distress i.e. use of accessory muscles, tracheal tug
   f Head tilt
      Chin lift
      Oropharyngeal airway
      Nasopharyngeal airway
      Laryngeal mask
      Endotracheal intubation
   g Cushing syndrome

The Monro–Kelly Doctrine describes the compensation mechanism in place to prevent a rise in intracranial pressure (ICP) following the development of an intracranial mass, such as a haematoma. The skull is essentially a container of a fixed volume. When a haematoma forms, cerebrospinal fluid and venous blood are squeezed out of the skull to ensure ICP stays constant. When this compensatory mechanism is exhausted, just a small increase in volume results in an exponential increase in ICP.

9 a An ankle X-ray is indicated if there is pain in either malleoli zones, and any of the below are present:
Bone tenderness on the posterior edge or tip of the lateral malleoli.
Bone tenderness on the posterior edge or tip of medial malleoli.
Inability to weight bear both immediately or in the casualty department.
A foot X-ray is required if there is any pain in the midfoot zone, and any of the below findings are present:
Bone tenderness on the base of 5th metatarsal.
Bone tenderness on the navicular.
Inability to weight bear both immediately or in the casualty department.

b Danis Weber/Lauge Hansen system

c Laterally: the anterior talofibular ligament, the calcaneofibular ligament, talofibular ligament
Medially: the deltoid ligament
Anterior: the anterior inferior tibiofibular ligament
Posterior: the posterior inferior tibiofibular ligament
The transverse ligaments

d USS/Duplex scan

e Therapeutic dose LMWH

Ottowa also developed a set of rules to determine whether an X-ray is required; an X-ray is required if a patient has suffered a knee injury and any of the below applies:
- aged 55 or over
- has isolated tenderness of the patella (with no other bony tenderness)
- tenderness at the head of the fibula
- inability to flex to 90°
- inability to weight bear immediately and in the casualty department

10 a Rheumatoid factor (to confirm diagnosis – positive in 70% of cases)
Anti-CCP
FBC (to rule out anaemia or infection/platelets also often elevated)
CRP/ESR (to check for any underlying infection or inflammation in the joints involved)

b Soft tissue swelling
Juxta articular osteopenia
Decreased joint space
Subluxation
Carpal destruction

c Nodules on the elbows and lungs
Lymphadenopathy

Vasculitis
Fibrosing alveolitis
Pleural and pericardial effusions
Raynaud's syndrome
CTS
Peripheral neuropathy
Splenomegaly

d Lifestyle aids with the help of occupational therapy
Regular exercise and physiotherapy
Suitable analgaesia such as paracetamol, codeine phosphate, ibuprofen or diclofenac (potentially with PPI cover)
Disease-modifying antirheumatic drugs (DMARDs) such as methotrexate, sulfasalazine, gold, penicillamine, azathioprine, anticytokine therapy.
Prednisolone
Biological agents such as infliximab.

Rheumatoid arthritis is a chronic systemic inflammatory disease, characterised by a usually symmetrical deforming peripheral polyarthritis. Classic deformities seen in the hand include swan neck or boutonniere deformities, Z deformity of thumb and MCP subluxation. The possibility of Atlantoaxial subluxation should also be remembered as this can threaten the spinal cord.

11 a Axillary nerve
b The 'regimental badge' region (lateral aspect of deltoid muscle)
c Anterior dislocation – caused by a fall onto an outstretched arm. Posterior dislocation – caused by forced internal rotation or blunt trauma to the anterior shoulder.
d IV morphine sulphate
Inhaled NO
IV midazolam
e Smith's fracture

Recurrent dislocation of the shoulder usually results from damage to the Glenoid Labrum and the subsequent formation of a pouch, the 'Bankart' lesion, into which the humeral head dislocates. Recurrence is commonest in the young (100-age = % recurrence rate). When aged >40 recurrence occurs in <10% of cases.

12 a Dupuytren's disease
     b Diabetes
         Epilepsy
         Trauma
         Alcoholism
         Smoking
         TB
         HIV
         Family history
         Age
         Female sex
     c Ring finger
     d Corticosteroid injection
     e Fasciectomy (removal of the thickened fascia)
         Fasciotomy (incision of the thickened fascia)

Dupytren's disease is a chronic progressive disease caused by the thickening and shortening of the palmar fascia and aponeurosis. Indications for surgery include a >30° fixed flexion at the MCP or PIP joints, or any particularly rapidly progressing contracture. The 'table top test' is used to determine the severity of the disease and extent of fixed deformities. Most patients with the disease do not require surgery.

13 a Septic arthritis
     b *Staphylococcus aureus*
         Streptococci
         Haemophilus influenza
         Neisseria gonorrhoea
         E. coli
     c FBC, U+Es, CRP
         Blood cultures
         X-ray of knee (AP and lateral)
         Microscopy, culture and sensitivity (MC+S)/microscopy and gram stain of an aspiration of synovial fluid from knee joint.
     d Benzylpenicillin
         Flucloxacillin
         Co-amoxiclav
     e Gout
         Pseudogout
         Trauma

Septic arthritis should be treated as a surgical emergency. The presence of bacteria and pus within a joint capsule can very quickly lead to the degeneration of hyaline cartilage which causes osteoarthritis. Patients should begin treatment with IV antibiotics, IV fluids, analgaesia, and if aspirates show significant infection, a surgical washout of the joint involved.

14 a Incision and drainage/surgical debridement
 b Diabetes
 IVDU (both causing immunosuppression)
 c Soft tissue swelling
 Patchy lucencies in the metaphyses.
 Periosteal new bone deformity.
 d *Staphylococcus aureus*
 Haemophilus influenza
 Streptococcus
 E. coli
 e Analgesia
 Bed rest
 Splint use
 IV antibiotics
 IV fluids
 Monitoring of fluid balance
 Surgical drainage of all mature subperiosteal abscesses
 Debridement of all necrotic tissue

Complications of acute OM include septicaemia, chronic OM, septic arthritis, and bony deformity (as a result of epiphyseal involvement). Chronic OM most commonly develops after open fractures or implanted metalwork become infected. It does sometimes develop however as a primary chronic infection of the bone i.e. TB.

15 a Tender anatomical snuff box
 Tender scaphoid tubercle
 Fullness in the snuff box (secondary to effusion)
 Painful wrist movements (particularly pronation followed by ulnar deviation)
 Pain on compression of the thumb longitudinally
 b Postero anterior (PA) wrist in ulnar deviation
 Lateral wrist in neutral
 PA in 45° pronation and ulnar deviation
 AP with 30° supination and ulnar deviation
 c The blood supply comes from distal perforating blood vessels therefore fractures cause decreased blood supply to the proximal portion leading to avascular necrosis.

d   Talus
    Head of femur
    Lunate (Kienbock's disease)
e   Early: bleeding, infection, anaesthetic risks, VTE
    Late: non-union, avascular necrosis, osteoarthritis

The scaphoid's blood supply runs from distal to proximal. As a result, the risk of non-union and avascular necrosis increases as the fracture site becomes more proximal. Management of non-displaced scaphoid waist fractures is conservative, with a below elbow cast used for 8 weeks. It should be noted that 12 weeks may be needed for complete fracture uniting to occur. Proximal or any displaced fractures require open reduction and internal fixation.

EMQs

1	**A**	10	**D**	19	**F**
2	**H**	11	**A**	20	**A**
3	**D**	12	**E**	21	**A**
4	**G**	13	**D**	22	**F**
5	**E**	14	**B**	23	**G**
6	**E**	15	**H**	24	**H**
7	**C**	16	**B**	25	**C**
8	**B**	17	**C**		
9	**A**	18	**D**		

MCQs

1   a – The Lauge Hansen and Weber classification systems concern ankle fractures. The Garden's system concerns intracapsular neck of femur fractures, whilst the Neer's system is used for humeral neck fractures.

2   c – The Thomson test involves lying the patient prone and squeezing their calf. Normally the foot moves as the ankle plantar flexes, but if the achilles has ruptured no movement will be seen.

3   b – Type I – the whole epiphysis is separated from the shaft, Type II – the epiphysis is displaced with a small triangular metaphyseal fragment (the commonest injury), Type III – separation of part of the epiphysis, Type IV – A separation of part of the epiphysis and metaphyseal fragment, Type V – Crushing of part, or all of the epiphyseal plate.

4   b – The radial nerve forms from the posterior cord of the brachial plexus. It has three main branches – the superficial branch, the deep branch, and the posterior cutaneous nerve of the forearm. The radial nerve provides motor distribution to the triceps, brachioradialis, extensor carpi radialis, supinator, extensor digitorum, extensor carpi ulnaris, abductor pollicis longus, extensor pollicis longus and brevis.

5   e – A locked knee, which is unequivocally caused by a meniscal injury, should be treated early with surgical intervention. Although swelling is common with peripheral meniscal tears, longitudinal tears may not result in an effusion. Joint line tenderness is the result of many knee injuries including meniscal tears. X-rays should always be performed to exclude bony injury.

6   e – The GCS scoring system is an objective measure of severity of brain injury. A GCS score of less than 8 is generally accepted as the definition of a coma or severe brain injury. A GCS of 9–12 suggests moderate brain injury, and 13–15 and minor brain injury. It is important to use the best motor response to stimulus when left/right asymmetry is present.

7   d – Bigelow's is a technique used to relocate a dislocated hip. Stimson's, Milch's, Kocher's and the Hippocratic technique are all ways to reduce a dislocated shoulder.

8   a – It is always important to assess the active and passive range of movements of a patient's joints on examination. Prior to this you should also inspect for any obvious deformity or swelling, and palpate for any tenderness, warmth or crepitus.

9   d – When fractured, the neck of femur, talus and scaphoid are all at significant risk of avascular necrosis. Non-union and delayed union are commonest in infected fractures, or if bone ends are not approximated exactly as a result of poor surgical technique or soft tissue interposition.

10 a – Congenital dislocation of the hip is usually evident at birth. The condition results from a defect in the superior acetabulum which results in a posterior dislocation. There are several theories as to why the condition occurs including abnormal intrauterine positioning, abnormal levels of maternal hormones or a genetic basis.

Chapter 7

Breast surgery

Gita S Patel

SAQs

1 A patient has had a recent lumpectomy and presents with a swelling at the scar site.

    a Give three potential causes for the swelling and provide a description of each. (6 marks)

    b The swelling is aspirated and colourless fluid obtained. What is the treatment of this condition? (1 mark)

    c Give three complications of treating this condition. (3 marks)

    d If yellow/green fluid is aspirated what investigation would you request and why? (2 marks)

2 An 18-year-old lady presents to you with asymmetrical breasts. She demands an operation to correct this.

    a What does mammoplasty mean? (1 mark)

    b Name three indications for mammoplasty. (3 marks)

    c Give two pieces of information you would convey to a patient, when obtaining their consent for surgery. (2 marks)

    d Name five risks of breast augmentation surgery. (5 marks)

3 A 53-year-old lady presents requesting advice on breast cancer as her friend has recently been diagnosed with the disease and she is worried.

    a Give three visible symptoms that a patient with non-metastasised breast cancer could initially present with. (3 marks)

    b Name five risk factors for developing breast cancer. (5 marks)

    c What is the staging system used for breast cancer? (1 mark)

    d What three methods of tumour spreading does this staging system assess? (3 marks)

    e Give two treatment modalities that are available for breast cancer. (2 marks)

4 A 60-year-old breast cancer patient undergoing treatment presents with new onset confusion.
  a Name four healthcare professionals who could be in the breast cancer MDT. (4 marks)
  b State two methods of breast cancer metastasis. (2 marks)
  c Name four body sites breast cancer is most likely to metastasise to. (4 marks)
  d State four things you would do if you had to tell someone their breast cancer had recurred. (4 marks)

5 A patient presents with mastitis of her left breast after 3 weeks of breast-feeding.
  a What is mastitis? (1 mark)
  b Give three signs of mastitis. (3 marks)
  c Give two potential causes for mastitis. (2 marks)
  d Can patients still breastfeed if they have mastitis? (1 mark)
  e State two blood tests you would do and explain why. (2 marks)
  f Give two treatment options available for this patient. (2 marks)

6 An 18-year-old girl presents with a lump in her right breast.
  a Give three specific questions you would ask in the history. (3 marks)
  b Give six details you should note about the lump on examination. (6 marks)
  c Name three of the differentials for the breast lump. (3 marks)

7 A 9-year-old girl presents with a lump that she felt deep to her left nipple.
  a What is the lump most likely to be? (1 mark)
  b What is the name of the period of puberty that includes breast development? (1 mark)
  c When does it occur during puberty? (1 mark)
  d State two other physical effects of puberty in a girl. (2 marks)
  e State three physical effects of puberty in a boy. (3 marks)
  f When examining breasts why do you palpate with the flat of the hand and not the fingertips? (2 marks)
  g When examining breasts why are the axillae included? (1 mark)

8 A 34-year-old lady presents with bilateral nipple discharge.
  a Give five questions you would ask in the history. (5 marks)
  b What is galactorrhoea? (1 mark)
  c Name two causes of galactorrhoea. (2 marks)
  d What initial investigation would you do? (1 mark)
  e What would you advise the patient if there are no abnormalities detected on investigation? (1 mark)

9 A 48-year-old woman would like some information on the breast screening programme.

    a Give four criteria that need to be fulfilled for a screening programme to be effective.   (4 marks)

    b Give three criteria for an adequate investigation method used in a screening programme.   (3 marks)

    c What is sensitivity?   (1 mark)

    d What is specificity?   (1 mark)

    e What is the age range for the UK breast screening programme?   (1 mark)

    f How often are women invited to attend for breast screening?   (1 mark)

    g What investigation method is used in the breast screening programme?   (1 mark)

    h Can you name another national screening programme for cancer?   (1 mark)

10 A 52-year-old woman is referred to a breast clinic under the 2 week wait scheme due to a palpable lump in the lower outer quadrant of her right breast.

    a What are the three modes of investigation used?   (3 marks)

    b Why is the screening programme investigation method less reliable in women less than 50 years old?   (1 mark)

    c Name two ways of taking cytology samples.   (2 marks)

    d Give two blood tests that are important to do specifically before a patient undergoes surgery.   (2 marks)

    e Give two investigations you would request if a patient known to have breast cancer presents with bone pain.   (2 marks)

    f What investigation would you do if a patient with known breast cancer presents with new onset confusion and all blood results are unchanged?   (1 mark)

EMQs

A patient presents with a breast lump.

A Seroma
B Abscess
C Haematoma
D Mastitis
E Fibroadenoma
F Breast cyst
G Breast bud
H Breast cancer

I Palpable lymph node
J Lipoma

1 A 33-year-old lady had a lumpectomy on her right breast 2 days ago and now the skin overlying the wound site looks bruised and feels hard and tender.
2 A 27-year-old lady with a 2 cm diameter lump on her left breast for as long as she can remember and she has had numerous similar lumps removed from her back and limbs.
3 A 35-year-old lady has been breastfeeding for 2 weeks now and her right breast has become hot, red and tender over the last 24 hours.
4 A 65-year-old lady with a lump in her left breast that has gradually increased in size over the last 4 months and is now changing the appearance of her skin.
5 A 7-year-old girl is seen with her mum due to a new lump that has appeared under her left nipple that is slightly tender.

Which investigation is the most appropriate?
A Mammography
B Ultrasound
C Fine needle aspiration cytology (FNAC)
D FBC
E Blood culture
F CT head scan
G Isotope bone scan
H Serum calcium
I LFTs
J U+Es
K Chest X-ray
L Clotting screen

6 A 59-year-old lady presents with a 2-week history of a palpable lump in her right breast.
7 A 43-year-old lady who underwent treatment for metastatic breast cancer presents to the emergency department with a 1 week history of increasing confusion.
8 A 54-year-old lady is admitted to the emergency department following a fall, and injury to her left forearm. On further questioning, she admits to have had gradually increasing generalised bone pain for the last few months.
9 A 26-year-old lady presents with a 1 cm diameter lump in her left breast that has been present for about 2 months.
10 A 45-year-old lady has had a wide local excision to her left breast 1 week ago and has presented to the emergency department with a fever, chills and rigors.

Match the description to the diagnosis:
A Fibrocystic disease
B Prolactinoma
C Paget's disease of the nipple
D Breast carcinoma
E Mammary duct ectasia
F Mammary duct fistula
G Lactation
H Intraductal papilloma

11 A 33-year-old lady presents with a 6-week history of a painless serous discharge from her right nipple. Examination is otherwise normal.
12 A 42-year-old lady presents with a brown discharge from both nipples, and tenderness in both breasts.
13 A 25-year-old lady presents with a white discharge from both nipples. She has also been having difficulty getting pregnant.
14 A 70-year-old presents with a blood stained discharge from the left nipple.
15 A 62-year-old lady presents with redness, scaling, and flaking of the skin of the nipple.

Match the appropriate treatment with the condition below:
A Incision and drainage
B Reassurance and analgesia
C Needle aspiration
D Antibiotics
E Mastectomy
F Surgical excision only
G Surgery with chemoradiotherapy

16 Non-infectious mastitis
17 Small breast abscess
18 Breast cancer
19 Ductal carcinoma *in situ*
20 Fibroadenoma

Please select the most appropriate answer from the list below:

A Paget's disease
B Core biopsy
C Pregnancy
D FNAC
E Lymph node involvement
F Breast cancer
G Fibrocystic disease
H Mastitis

21 A 20-year-old lady with a small moveable rubbery breast lump is seen in the breast clinic. She has an examination and ultrasound. What further investigation is required?
22 A 57-year-old lady has excision of a breast cancer for a presumed non-metastatic lump. What feature histologically suggests a worse prognosis?
23 A 70-year-old lady has a discoloration with roughness on her left nipple, which is not resolving with cream. What is the likely diagnosis?
24 What is the most common cause of breast lumps in a woman under the age of 30?
25 A 24-year-old lady presents with bilateral heavy uncomfortable breasts which have become more lumpy with dilated veins over the last 2 months.

MCQs

1 If the breast screening programme was trialling a decrease in minimum age to 40, and the number of false positive and true positive results increased which statistical value would increase?
   a Sensitivity
   b Specificity
   c Negative predictive value
   d Positive predictive value
   e Prevalence

2 Which dermatome innervates the nipple?
   a T2
   b T3
   c T4
   d T5
   e T6

3 Which of the following is not a risk factor for breast cancer?
   a   Early menopause
   b   Early menarche
   c   Positive family history
   d   Nulliparity
   e   Contraceptive pill

4 A 20-year-old girl comes to see you with a lump in her left breast. It is small, mobile, and difficult to pin down. What is the most likely diagnosis?
   a   Breast carcinoma
   b   Breast abscess
   c   Fibroadenoma
   d   Lipoma
   e   Fat necrosis

5 Which of the following is not associated with gynaecomastia?
   a   Liver failure
   b   Renal failure
   c   Spironolactone
   d   Hyperthyroidism
   e   Congestive cardiac failure

6 A breast tumour is found to have a TNM stage of T3N1M0. Which of the following statements is true regarding this staging?
   a   The tumour has metastasised
   b   The ipsilateral lymph nodes are involved
   c   The tumour is between 2 cm and 5 cm diameter
   d   The tumour has invaded the chest wall
   e   There are supraclavicular lymph nodes involved

7 Milk secretion is stimulated by which hormone?
   a   Luteinising hormone (LH)
   b   Dopamine
   c   Oestrogen
   d   Prolactin
   e   Follicle stimulating hormone (FSH)

8 Which of the following is not a complication of breast reduction surgery?
   a   Loss of areola sensation
   b   Difficulty breastfeeding
   c   Infection
   d   Nipple discharge
   e   Bleeding

9 Which of the following patients would be permitted breast augmentation on the NHS?

   a   A 17-year-old girl who is depressed as she feels that no one is attracted to her due to small breasts

   b   A 23-year-old lady who is 4 months pregnant, and has severe breast asymmetry

   c   A 55-year-old lady who had a right mastectomy due to breast cancer

   d   A 53-year-old lady with breast cancer who has not yet finished chemotherapy

10 Which of the following signs or symptoms is not associated with a simple breast cyst?

   a   A smooth round breast lump which is moveable

   b   Increased lump size prior to menstruation

   c   Cyclical breast pain

   d   Improvement of symptoms following menstruation

   e   Skin changes overlying the lump

Answers

SAQs

1 **a** Abscess – a pus-filled lesion enclosed in a membrane
Seroma – an accumulation of serous fluid
Haematoma – an accumulation of blood
Mastitis – inflammation of the breast tissue, which may or may not
have an infective cause

b Drainage of the seroma by aspiration

c Pain
Bleeding
Infection
Scar
Recurrence

d Microscopy, culture and sensitivity of the aspirated fluid.
To determine the causative organism, and an appropriate antibiotic
to prescribe if indicated.

Patients should be warned about the risks of surgery in order to gain
valid consent for the procedure. The commonest side-effects should
be explained as well as the most serious, with the symptoms made clear
so that the patient can present early if required. Patients should also be
warned that although these side-effects such as seroma and abscess can be
treated they may recur.

2 **a** Reconstruction of a breast.

b Correction of breast defects – e.g. congenital abnormalities, effects
of trauma, breast diseases such as cancer.
Revision of previous breast surgery such as a mastectomy.
Patient's choice based on expected psychological benefits.

c An explanation of the surgical procedure.
The indication for the procedure.
Explanation of the possible risks.
Explanation of the possible benefits.

d Pain/altered sensation
Infection/abscess formation
Bleeding/haematoma formation
Seroma formation
Asymmetry
Scar formation

Injury to surrounding structures e.g. nerves
Failure of procedure
Breastfeeding problems
Anaesthetic complications

As with any surgery, it is important to outline the risks and benefits in a way the patient can understand. They should then be given adequate time to decide on whether they still want to proceed. Patients can withdraw their consent for surgery at any point pre-operatively. It should be made clear to patients that although they should be able to breastfeed after a mammoplasty operation they may have difficulties with this due to the surgery.

3 a A breast lump
          Peau d'orange around the nipple
          Erythema around the nipple
          Scaling around the nipple
          Blood-stained discharge from the nipple
          An inverted nipple
          Fungating lesion
          Weight loss
     b Female gender
          Early menarche
          Nulliparity
          Female older than 30 years before their first child is born.
          Late menopause
          Previous breast cancer
          Previous ovarian cancer
          Previous endometrial cancer
          Family history of breast cancer
     c TNM staging
     d Spread to lymph nodes
          Metastatic spread
     e Surgery
          Chemotherapy
          Radiotherapy
          Hormone treatment

Breast cancer is the commonest female malignancy in the UK. Breast cancer awareness is widespread and many patients will present concerning this. It is important to educate patients on the correct facts about the condition and the process from diagnosis to treatment. If a patient is suspected to have breast cancer they should be referred to a specialist breast clinic on the 2-week wait system. The management plan should be devised in negotiation with the patient and a multi-disciplinary team in order to create the best treatment plan for each individual patient.

4   a   Breast surgeon
            Breast care nurse
            Oncologist
            Radiologist
            Pathologist
            Clinical psychologist
            Plastic surgeon
      b   Direct local extension
            Lymphatics
            Blood vessels
      c   Skin
            Nearby lymph nodes
            Contralateral breast
            Bones
            Lungs
            Brain
            Ovaries
            Liver
      d   Ensure there is adequate time, privacy, and space, with appropriate family and team members present.
            Allow their family and/or friends to be present if the patient wants them there.
            Have all the information at hand.
            Find out what they already know and how much information they would like.
            Give a warning shot.
            Provide written information on everything that is discussed.
            Offer a follow up appointment.

Patients require adequate psychological support in addition to the therapeutic or palliative management of their breast cancer. This can enable them to participate in the decision-making process for their management. There are a number of support networks for cancer patients and these should be highlighted. Patients and their carers should be warned about the risks of metastases and the symptoms they should be looking out for in order to present as early as possible.

5 a It is an inflammation of the breast tissue. It can be infective or non-infective.

    b Rubor – redness
Calor – warm
Dolor – painful
Tumour – swollen

    c Milk stasis (i.e. blocked duct causing inflammation through local pressure effects)
Skin trauma (i.e. cracked nipples allowing infection to penetrate through to the breast tissue)

    d Yes (if the patient can tolerate the pain, it is beneficial to feed more often from the affected breast)

    e FBC – to check for a raised white cell count and neutrophil count
Blood culture – to check for infective organisms in the blood stream

    f A course of antibiotics, if the mastitis is more likely to be infective.
Conservative management, with analgesia and anti-pyretics as necessary, if infection is unlikely.

There are five cardinal signs of inflammation. These are tumour (swelling), dolor (pain), calor (increased temperature), rubor (erythema), and function leasa (loss of function). Symptomatic treatment (including anti-pyretics and analgesia) should always be advised in addition to targeted therapy in order to regain function as soon as possible.

6 a When did the lump appear?
Has it changed in any way since it first appeared?
Is there any discharge from it?
Was there a trigger?
Is there any pain or an altered sensation?
Do your periods have any effect on it?
Have you used any topical creams/ointments on it?
Do you have any other lumps?
Family history of breast cancer?
Obstetric history

    b Site
Size
Surface
Shape
Edge
Colour
Consistency
What it is attached to (e.g. skin or muscle)?

Can it be moved?
Does it fluctuate?
Does it transilluminate?
Does it have any discharge?

c   Lipoma
Sebaceous cyst
Enlarged lymph node
Breast cyst
Fibroadenoma
Cancer

It is important to take any patient presenting with a breast lump very seriously as they all have the same underlying concern; is this lump a cancer? The same basic history and examination should be performed for all and referral made to the breast clinic if clinically appropriate. Statistically, the younger a patient the more likely it is that the lump will be benign but it is vital to remember that young women get breast cancer too.

7 a   A breast bud
b   Thelarche
c   First stage of puberty
d   Pubic hair growth
Axillary hair growth
Increased subcutaneous fat deposition around the hips
Menarche
e   Enlargement of genitalia
Pubic hair growth
Axillary hair growth
Facial hair growth
Voice becomes deeper
f   There is a lot of fatty tissue in breasts especially in younger women and this can feel lumpy when palpating with your fingertips which are highly sensitive.
g   The tail of the breast tissue rises up to the axilla and axillary lymph nodes can also be palpated.

Many girls present with breast bud formation. The left breast bud commonly develops before the right breast bud and the asymmetry of development and associated tenderness can worry some patients. These patients should be reassured that this is a normal process of development and be provided with adequate verbal and written information to allay their concerns.

8 **a** What is the discharge like? (colour/consistency)
When did the discharge start?
Is it constant?
Did anything trigger it?
Has the discharge changed?
Have you noticed any other breast changes?
When was your last period?
Could you be pregnant?
Are you taking any medications or herbal supplements?

b Discharge of milk from a breast that is not due to breastfeeding.

c Hyperprolactinaemia
Physical stimulation of the breasts
Medications e.g. selective serotonin re-uptake inhibitors

d Serum prolactin level – probable hyperprolactinaemia if >500 mU/L

e To try to prevent any physical stimulation of their breasts.

Galactorrhoea may be due to hyperprolactinaemia, other symptoms of which are breast pain, infertility, oligomenorrhoea and amenorrhoea. MRI head may demonstrate a prolactinoma which is a prolactin secreting tumour (usually a pituitary adenoma). Dopamine agonists such as bromocriptine and cabergoline are used to inhibit prolactin secretion medically although if this does not work trans-sphenoidal resection may be required.

9 **a** The condition being screened for should be significant within the population screened.
It should be possible to diagnose the condition at an early stage.
The investigation method used should be acceptable to the screened population.
The investigation method used should have a high specificity.
The investigation method used should have a high sensitivity.
There should be adequate facilities for both diagnosis and treatment.
The treatment offered for the diagnosed condition should be acceptable to the screened population.
The screening programme as a whole, should be cost-effective.

b Acceptable to the screened population
Can be replicated
High sensitivity
High specificity
Relatively easy to perform and interpret

c   Sensitivity is the proportion of true positives that are correctly identified by the investigation method. For example, the proportion of patients that have early breast cancer that are diagnosed by the breast screening programme.

d   Specificity is the proportion of true negatives that are correctly identified by the investigation method. For example, the proportion of healthy patients, not diagnosed with breast cancer by the breast screening programme.

e   50–70 years old

f   Every 3 years

g   Mammography

h   Cervical screening programme
     Bowel cancer screening programme

The breast screening programme is for women aged 50–70 years old that are asymptomatic, in order to diagnose and subsequently treat breast cancer early. If a woman presents with symptoms that could lead to a clinical diagnosis of possible breast cancer then she should be referred under the 2-week wait scheme to a specialist breast clinic. The risks of a screening programme are the false negatives and false positives, and these should be minimised for an effective screening programme. The breast screening programme also subjects the population screened to X-ray radiation every 3 years but studies have shown that the risks of the radiation are outweighed by the possibility of detecting breast cancer early.

10 a   Mammography
        Ultrasound
        Biopsy

    b   Their breasts are denser due to the increased volume of fatty tissue so there is more likelihood of false positives.

    c   FNAC
         Core biopsy
         Open biopsy

    d   Clotting screen
         Group and save sample
         FBC (this could reveal anaemia that requires a transfusion and/or an infection)
         U+Es (very abnormal results will need to be corrected before surgery, and will direct fluid management in the peri-operative period)

    e   Serum calcium
         Isotope bone scan
         X-ray of the site of the pain

    f   CT head scan

The diagnosis of breast cancer should be based on clinical suspicion, from the history and examination, and the results of investigations. The patient should be counselled on each investigation and the importance of the results in the clinical context in order to increase compliance and reduce anxiety. Patients should be discussed at the local MDT to ensure appropriate investigations and treatment are carried out.

EMQs

1	**C**	10	**E**	19	**E**
2	**J**	11	**E**	20	**F**
3	**D**	12	**A**	21	**D**
4	**H**	13	**B**	22	**E**
5	**G**	14	**D**	23	**A**
6	**A**	15	**C**	24	**G**
7	**F**	16	**B**	25	**C**
8	**G**	17	**C**		
9	**C**	18	**G**		

MCQs

1   a

	Patient with breast cancer	Healthy patient
Test positive	True positive	False positive
Test negative	False negative	True negative

Positive predictive value = True positive/ (True positive + False positive) × 100.

Negative predictive value = True negative/ (True negative +False negative) × 100.

Sensitivity = True positive/ (True positive + False negative) × 100

Specificity = True negative/ (True negative + False positive) × 100.

2   c – The breasts are innervated by the 3rd to 5th thoracic dermatomes, with the nipple innervated largely by the lateral cutaneous branch of T4.

3   a – There are several factors which increase the risk of breast cancer, including age, female, BRCA1, BRCA2, family history, personal history, Caucasian, early menarche, late menopause, radiation exposure, nulliparity, first child after 30 years, COCP, HRT, alcohol, and obesity.

4 c – A fibroadenoma is a benign breast tumour which is usually firm, rubbery, painless, and easily movable.

5 e – Gynaecomastia is an enlargement of male breast tissue, caused by a lack of testosterone, excess of oestrogen, and a variety of medications.

6 b – T3 is a tumour greater than 5 cm diameter, N1 has affected the upper level of lymph nodes in the axilla, M0 described no distant metastases.

7 d – Prolactin is released by the anterior pituitary gland due to stimulation of the nipple during breast feeding, stimulating milk production and secretion.

8 d – Nipple discharge is not expected following mammoplasty.

9 c – Breast augmentation is usually only funded by the NHS in cases where there is complete breast agenesis, severe asymmetry, or post-tumour excision. It should not be done in any patient under 18, during pregnancy, prior to tumour excision, or if any infection is present.

10 e – Overlying skin changes are a sign of malignancy.

Chapter 8

Paediatric surgery

Shafiq Arif Shahban

SAQs

1 A 6-week-old boy is taken to A&E by his mother who says he is vomiting after feeds.

    a What four further questions would you like to ask about the vomiting to help in making a diagnosis?   (4 marks)

    b You suspect pyloric stenosis, list three other differential diagnoses.   (3 marks)

    c What biochemical derangement fits with the diagnosis of pyloric stenosis?   (3 marks)

    d What would be your initial management at this stage? List three points.   (3 marks)

    e Name the surgical procedure which can correct this diagnosis.   (1 mark)

2 An 8-month-old boy who is crying persistently is brought to the emergency department.

    a Define inconsolable crying.   (1 mark)

    b On further questioning, you ascertain that his crying is episodic and that when he does cry he draws up his legs, and occasionally vomits. List three differential diagnoses.   (3 marks)

    c The father tells you that his son has, on occasions, passed stools which are redcurrant coloured. What is the most likely diagnosis?   (1 mark)

    d What is the investigation of choice and what is the name of the sign consistent with this diagnosis?   (2 marks)

    e Give three aspects of your initial management.   (3 marks)

3 A 1-month-old boy is admitted to the paediatric ward with his concerned parents who have noticed a lump on his abdomen.

    a Give four further questions you would like to ask the parents regarding the lump. (4 marks)

    b Excluding size and location, list four features to comment on when examining a lump. (4 marks)

    c On examining the child, you find a 2 cm × 2 cm swelling in the umbilical area. You suspect this is an umbilical hernia, list two further differential diagnoses. (2 marks)

    d Define a hernia. (2 marks)

    e What differentiates a primary hernia from a secondary hernia? (2 marks)

4 You are the doctor on the delivery suite and on examining a premature newborn find him to have only one testicle.

    a You suspect that he has an undescended testicle, give three other possible causes for this finding. (3 marks)

    b Briefly describe the path taken for the normal descent of a testicle *in utero*. (3 marks)

    c List one advantage of having the testicles lie in the scrotal sac outside of the abdominal cavity. (1 mark)

    d List one possible complication of one or both testicles remaining in the abdominal cavity instead of the scrotal sac. (1 mark)

    e Briefly describe the management options for this undescended testicle. (2 marks)

5 A 4-year-old boy is taken to his GP by his mother, who tells you that she is worried about his penile skin which does not retract.

    a Define phimosis and paraphimosis. (2 marks)

    b List four questions to ask at this stage. (4 marks)

    c On examination of his penile skin, you notice a white discharge. List two appropriate steps with regards to his management. (2 marks)

    d Give one non-surgical method to help to release phimosis and paraphimosis. (1 mark)

    e Which surgical procedure is used to treat phimosis? (1 mark)

6 Mrs R is a young lady who is pregnant for the 1st time, and at her 20 week antenatal USS she is told that she has a raised alpha fetaprotein (AFP) level and also that the USS shows that her child has gastroschisis.

    a What is gastroschisis? (2 marks)

    b AFP is one components of the 'triple test', list the two other components to this test. (2 marks)

    c   List two additional precautions which will be made for
this patient's pregnancy.   (2 marks)

    d   Describe two possible complications for the child if the
abdominal contents were not adequately covered at the
time of delivery.   (2 marks)

    e   Soon after birth this child has corrective surgery to
restore the abdominal contents to the abdominal cavity.
List two measures to be taken post-operatively.   (2 marks)

7   Tommy is 2-years-old, and after a fall from playing in the garden he
complains of pain in his right arm. An X-ray of this region shows a
Salter–Harris Class III fracture of the right humerus.

    a   Name two other types of fracture.   (2 marks)

    b   Describe what is meant by Salter–Harris Class III
fracture.   (2 marks)

    c   Name and differentiate between the cells which help to
form bone from those which break down bone.   (2 marks)

    d   You see this child in A&E. After requesting and
reporting on the X-ray, list three further steps in the
management of Tommy.   (3 marks)

    e   Tommy has his fracture treated conservatively. With
specific regard to this fracture type, list one possible
complication.   (1 mark)

8   You see a baby for her 6-week baby check. On examination of the hips,
you suspect that she has developmental dysplasia of the hips (DDH).

    a   Give two questions you would like to ask the parents to
help you to reach this diagnosis.   (2 marks)

    b   Name two clinical tests used to help to diagnose DDH.   (2 marks)

    c   List two non-invasive investigations you would like to
order at this stage.   (2 marks)

    d   List two treatment options for this patient.   (2 marks)

    e   The baby has an operation to correct her DDH. List
two specific complications for this operation.   (2 marks)

9   A 6-year-old boy is taken to his GP with hearing problems.

    a   You are concerned that he may have glue ear. List three
alternative differential diagnoses.   (3 marks)

    b   What is the medical term for glue ear?   (1 mark)

    c   To help you to make a diagnosis of glue ear what further
questions would you like to ask?   (2 marks)

    d   You strongly suspect he has glue ear. What management
would you initiate?   (3 marks)

    e   This child's glue ear is treated with grommets. Explain
how these help.   (2 marks)

10 You see James in A&E, a 12-year-old boy, who complains of intense bilateral knee pain, which has been on and off for a month, but slowly getting worse over the past 4 days. At this moment, you are thinking that James may have Osgood-Schlatter disease.

    a List two further differential diagnoses. (2 marks)

    b Give three tests you would like to request to differentiate between these diagnoses. (3 marks)

    c List two non-surgical methods of treatment. (2 marks)

    d The non-surgical methods fail to help James and so he is to have corrective surgery. You are the junior doctor on the paediatric surgical ward. List four things you would ensure with regards to his pre-op preparation. (4 marks)

EMQs

Match the diagnosis to the descriptions:

A Slipped upper femoral epiphysis
B Perthes disease
C Juvenile arthritis
D Talipes equinovarus
E Tubular arthritis
F Osgood-Schlatter disease
G Septic arthritis

1 Congenital condition consisting of foot inversion and plantar flexion.
2 Symptoms include joint pain and tenderness and feeling systemically unwell.
3 Arthritis of one or more joints in patients less than 18 years-of-age.
4 Growth plate swelling and tenderness at the tibial tuberosity.
5 Fracture through the growth plate of the femoral physis.
6 Infection of the joint caused by a type of acid fast bacilli.
7 Idiopathic avascular necrosis of the femoral head.

Match the fluid deficit to the correct patient:

A 1800 ml
B 50 ml
C 375 ml
D 300 ml
E 750 ml

8 7.5 kg child with 10% dehydration.
9 7.5 kg child with 5% dehydration.

10 12 kg child with 15% dehydration.
11 6 kg child with 5% dehydration.
12 0.5 kg child with 10% dehydration.

Match the diagnosis to the description:
A Testicular torsion
B Hydrocoele
C Haematocoele
D Epididymal cyst
E Maldescended testicle
F Hernia

13 A 2-year-old boy is admitted with a markedly swollen uncomfortable left testicle. It has been slightly swollen for several months, but recently got worse. On examination, it is transilluminating brilliantly.
14 A 16-year-old boy with a sudden onset of pain in the right testicle of 6 hours duration. It is painful to walk or sit. There is no history of trauma.
15 A 6-week-old baby is seen by the GP for the 6-week check. The left testicle feels normal, however he is unable to feel the right.

Match the description to the diagnosis:
A Otitis media
B Otitis externa
C Perforated drum
D Glue ear
E Vestibular neuritis
F Impacted wax

16 A 6-year-old boy is seen in clinic. His teacher says that he often seems distracted, and finds it difficult to follow instructions, when he was previously bright.
17 A complication of using cotton buds.
18 A 12-year-old girl with pain in her left ear. On examination, there is a red bulging drum, and the hearing is reduced unilaterally.

Match the diagnosis to the description:

A Intersussception
B Appendicitis
C Bowel obstruction
D Mesenteric adenitis
E Hirschsprung's disease
F Pyloric stenosis
G GORD

19 Classically, parents describe their children as having projectile vomiting shortly after feeding, and on examination you may palpate a pyloric mass.
20 Patients often complain of abdominal pain following a recent viral infection.
21 The child, usually aged 2–24 months, has colicky abdominal pain and can often pass redcurrant jelly stools.
22 This can be treated surgically using Nissen's funduplication procedure.
23 Classically, this occurs during the early teenage years and patients complain of pain over McBurney's point, and they may also be Rovsing's Sign positive.
24 Congenital absence of ganglionic cells within the anus
25 Patients often complain of abdominal distension, bilious vomiting, and constipation.

MCQs

1 In A&E you see a child who has a 1-day history of persistent diarrhoea and gastroenteritis. He weighs 8.2 kg and is thought to be 5% dehydrated based on clinical examination. What is this child's fluid deficit?
  a   320 ml
  b   410 ml
  c   500 ml
  d   120 ml
  e   630 ml

2 You see a child on the paediatric ward who weighs 17 kg, and as the junior doctor you are asked to calculate their maintenance fluids. What is this child's maintenance fluid requirement over 24 hours?
  a   1050 ml
  b   1150 ml
  c   1250 ml
  d   1350 ml
  e   1450 ml

3 You are called to see a young child in the resus area of A&E who has stridor. Which of the following is the most likely cause?
a Asthma
b Foreign body aspiration
c Pneumonia
d Bronchiolitis
e Swine flu

4 In A&E you see a 14-year-old boy who complains of intense pain in the scrotal area of 3 hours duration, and on examination, you notice that the scrotum is swollen and the testicle retracted. What is the most likely diagnosis?
a Testicular torsion
b Inguinal hernia
c Epididymitis
d Hydrocele
e Variocele

5 Cleft lip is a physical abnormality which can often be detected antenatally, how many cases of this condition are reported, per 1000?
a 1
b 10
c 15
d 20
e 50

6 A 5-year-old boy has a fracture through the growth plate metaphysis only. Please identify the correct type of fracture.
a Salter-Harris I
b Salter-Harris II
c Salter-Harris III
d Salter-Harris IV
e Salter-Harris V

7 Which of the following allows blood to bypass the liver *in utero*?
a Ductus arteriosus
b Umbilical vein
c Foramen ovale
d Ductus venosus
e Umbilical artery

8 Duodenal atresia is associated with which genetic condition?
   a   Klinefelter
   b   Gaucher's disease
   c   Down syndrome
   d   Edwards syndrome
   e   Patau syndrome

9 A 4-week-old baby is brought to see you with a large raised dimpled red lesion on the face.
   a   Infantile haemangioma
   b   Café au lait spot
   c   Mongolian blue spot
   d   Port wine stain
   e   Telangiectatic naevus

10 A 1-year-old is admitted with burns to the whole of both lower legs after being placed in a very hot bath. The percentage of body surface area burnt is?
   a   25%
   b   20%
   c   18%
   d   15%
   e   10%

Answers

SAQs

1 a Is the vomit projectile?
What colour is the vomit?
Is there associated diarrhoea?
How much does he bring up?
How long after the feed does he vomit?
Is this something new or has this been happening since birth?
Is there or has there ever been blood in the vomit?

  b GORD
Gastroenteritis
Milk posseting/overfeeding

  c Hypochloraemic
Hypokalaemic
Metabolic acidosis

  d NBM
Bloods – FBC, U+E, LFTs, CRP
Cannulate and give IV fluids
Consider arranging USS

  e Ramstedt's pyloromyotomy

Pyloric stenosis typically occurs between 6 and 8 weeks of age, males are affected four times more than females. The diagnosis is largely clinical, however USS may be required. Parents describe that their child has projectile vomiting after every feed. Children become malnourished and dehydrated, therefore, IV fluids are necessary.

2 a Unresponsive and prolonged crying episodes in a toddler/infant.

  b Bowel intussusception
Umbilical hernia
Colic
Gastroenteritis
Teething

  c Bowel intussusception

  d USS
Donut sign

  e NBM
Analgesia
Bloods (FBC, CRP, U+E, LFT, G+S)
IV fluids

Intussusception typically occurs between 6 and 12 months, but can present in toddlers and rarely older patients. In addition to the above findings it may be possible to palpate a sausage-shaped abdominal mass. In severe cases, patients can present with shock. Management is often conservative, however treatment may require administration of an air or barium enema. If this fails then surgical intervention is required. In all cases there is a roughly 5% recurrence rate.

3 a When did you first notice the lump?
Has the lump changed from when they first noticed it?
Does anything make the lump larger or smaller (such as coughing, sneezing or straining)?
Does the lump cause any distress to the child?
Have the parents noticed any lumps anywhere else?
Is the lump red?
Is the lump tender?

b Shape
Colour
Consistency
Contours
Temperature
Transillumination
Punctum/discharge
Mobile/fixed
Tender
Hot

c Paraumbilical hernia
Gastroschisis
Omphalocoele

d A hernia is an abnormal protrusion of part or all of the abdominal contents through a defect in the wall of the cavity in which it normally lies.

e A primary hernia is a natural occurrence of a hernia which can either be congenital or acquired. A secondary hernia describes herniation (often of bowels) through a surgical scar.

Umbilical hernias commonly occur shortly after birth as a result of a persistent defect in the overlying abdominal fascia. They are often not painful as the borders of the defect in the cavity wall are often large and can accommodate for this. In most children true umbilical hernias resolve spontaneously at around 4 years-of-age, very few children require surgical intervention.

4 a Poor positioning of the second testicle and missing feeling for it. Difference in size of the testicles.
Testicular agenesis.

b At around month 4 of gestation the testicle passes through the internal ring, the inguinal canal and the external ring, to take its final resting position in the scrotum.

c This allows for regulation and maintenance of the correct temperature for sperm production and thus fertility.

d There is a higher risk of testicular malignancy in this scenario. Increased risk of testicular torsion.

e Conservative management – do nothing, as the testicle may descend to the scrotum spontaneously
Surgical management – this depends on whether or not the testicle can be palpated, where it is located, and the age of the patient

Undescended testes are commoner in preterm babies than full-term babies and is typically a unilateral problem (although it can be bilateral). Diagnosis of this condition is largely clinical, however it can be confirmed by USS. It is more common in certain genetic conditions such as Prader-Willi syndrome or Kallman's syndrome. With an undescended testicle there is a 20% higher risk of that individual developing testicular malignancy and thus intervention is required.

5 a Phimosis – tight penile foreskin (prepuce) which is unable to be retracted behind the glans penis
Paraphimosis – tight penile foreskin around the penile shaft. which cannot be brought back into its normal position

b Does this cause any pain/discomfort for him?
Has she noticed any discharge?
Has he been seen to have a temperature or feel feverish?
Does this affect him when voiding?
Has it always been like this or has this happened only recently?
How did she come to notice it?
Is there any ballooning when he urinates?

c Swab and send sample for MC&S
Refer to urologists

d Topical steroid cream

e Circumcision

In phimosis the patient's foreskin is too tight which causes pain, redness, inflammation and even balinitis. Prior to the age of 4 it is normal to have non-retractile foreskin, but beyond this circumcision is often the treatment of choice. A second-line option is the use of steroid cream to help to reduce inflammation and therefore the symptoms.

6   a   Gastroschisis is the failure of closure of the anterior abdominal wall, thus allowing the persistent herniation of abdominal organs.

    b   β-HCG

    c   Involvement of paediatric surgeons
Involvement of neonatologists
Regular ultrasound monitoring for fetal growth
Antenatal counselling

    d   Increased risk of infection
Increased risk of heat loss, and thus hypothermia
Increased risk of water loss, and thus dehydration
Increased risk of bowel damage

    e   Transfer to neonatal intensive care unit (NICU) or special care baby unit (SCBU).
Regular observations of vital signs
Reassurance to the parents
Wound care

Gastroschisis is a rare but potentially fatal condition although corrective surgery has a 90% success rate. The biggest threat with this condition is the risk of infection, and thus it is vital to ensure that exposure to air is minimised, which may require paralysing and intubating at birth.

7   a   Open
Comminuted
Oblique
Spira
Transverse
Stress
Greenstick

    b   A complete fracture involving the bone, the epiphysis, the metaphysis, and the growth plate.

    c   Osteoblasts – cells involved in bone formation
Osteoclasts – cells involved in bone destruction

    d   Orthopaedic review
Analgesia
Fracture stabilisation
Ask about other injuries that may have been sustained from this event.
Reassurance for the parents.

    e   Stunted bone growth – as a result of growth plate involvement

Orthopaedic injuries in children are common, and can range from being simple to life-threatening. A typical fracture like this heals in 4–6 weeks without requiring surgical intervention. Greenstick fractures are a common type of fracture in children.

8 a Is there a family history of DDH?
Is this the first child?
Was the baby a breech presentation?
Was the baby delivered prematurely?

  b Barlow test
Ortolani test

  c USS
X-ray

  d Non-surgical – bracing (Pavlik harness) – this helps to keep the hip stable
Surgical – this is often used for slightly older children, or if the conservative methods fail to stabilise the hips

  e Avascular necrosis to the femoral head
Re-dislocation post procedure
Joint stiffness
Juvenile hip arthritis

DDH may be missed in the baby check, especially if performed by an inexperienced clinician. In older children there may be a history of delayed walking, waddling gait or pain. If hips are thought to be 'clicky' at birth, USS and orthopaedic referral should be arranged. DDH occurs more frequently in first born babies, premature babies and if there is a strong family history of DDH.

9 a Otitis externa
Foreign body within ear canal
Loud noise exposure
Trauma to the tympanic membrane

  b Otitis media with effusion

  c Does he suffer with recurrent ear infections?
Is his poor hearing something new, or is this the first time that this has been noticed?
Any discharge from the ear?
How is he getting on at school? Has there been a recent deterioration?

  d ENT referral
Audiogram
Tympanogram
Swab the ear canal and send for MC&S
Reassurance for the mother

e   A grommet is a device that sits in the tympanic membrane which allows for fluid which may have collected in the middle ear to be drained, and thus allowing for adequate tympanic membrane vibration and ultimately sound conduction.

Glue ear is very common in children. They have eustachian tubes which are short and straight allowing for ease of transmission for infection and difficulty in drainage. The pus that collects in the middle ear is what we refer to as glue ear, and unfortunately decongestants and mucolytic agents have little or no effect. In addition to grommet insertion, if severe enough, some children have adenoidectomies which helps by allowing for ease of drainage through the eustachian tube.

10 a   Septic arthritis
        Juvenile arthritis
        Soft tissue injury
        Transient synovitis
   b   FBC
        X-ray
        CRP
        Blood culture
        Joint aspiration
   c   Rest
        Analgesia
        Anti-inflammatory medication
        Ice compression to reduce swelling
   d   Cannula
        NBM
        Consent form completed
        Fluids prescribed
        Marked limb

Osgood–Schlatter disease, otherwise known as tibial tuberosity apophysitis, is commonest amongst 10–15-year-olds. It often presents as sharp knee pain which is worse on exercise. It is more common in males, and diagnosis is largely clinical. Management typically involves analgesia, anti-inflammatory medication and rest. Surgical treatment may be offered but this exposes the patient to significant risks.

EMQs

1	**D**	10	**A**	19	**F**
2	**G**	11	**D**	20	**D**
3	**C**	12	**B**	21	**A**
4	**F**	13	**B**	22	**G**
5	**A**	14	**A**	23	**B**
6	**E**	15	**E**	24	**E**
7	**B**	16	**D**	25	**C**
8	**E**	17	**F**		
9	**C**	18	**A**		

MCQs

1 b – Fluid deficit in children is calculated by the following formula:
Fluid deficit = weight (kg) × percentage dehydration × 10 ml.

2 d – Maintenance fluids in children are calculated using the following protocol:
100 ml/kg for the 1st 10 kg
50 ml/kg for the 2nd 10 kg
20 ml/kg for the remainder.
We are told that this child weighs 17 kg, and therefore 100 ml × 10 = 1000, and 50 ml × 7 = 350, giving us a total of 1350 ml over 24 hours.

3 b – Stridor is a high pitched musical sound, produced by obstruction along the upper airway respiratory tract, and thus a large foreign body aspiration is likely to get stuck and produce this sound. This is important to remember as a differential diagnosis in young children as this can occlude the airways and become fatal and may even require cricothyroidotomy.

4 a – Testicular torsion is a urological emergency and is common in adolescent boys. Early surgical intervention can save the testicle, however if left untreated the involved testicle can undergo avascular necrosis.

5 a – This condition occurs in 1 in 1000 infants and its management is multi-disciplinary. It can be picked up by USS antenatally. Many infants who have cleft lip also have cleft palate, and it is thus important to examine for this. Surgical repair of this condition usually take place after 3 months of age.

6 b – Type I is through the growth plate, type 2 through the growth plate and metaphysis, type 3 through the growth plate and epiphysis, type 4 through the growth plate metaphysis and epiphysis, and type 5 is a compression of the growth plate.

7   d – *In utero* blood enters through the umbilical vein, and then enters the ductus venosus which carries blood to the inferior vena cava. This leads to the right atrium, and blood passes from here through the foramen ovale to the left atrium, then around the body, and to the umbilical artery.

8   c – 20–40% of patients with duodenal atresia suffer with Down syndrome, with 8% of all patients with Down syndrome having duodenal atresia.

9   a – An infantile haemangioma or strawberry naevus occurs in 3–5% of babies. They may grow up until the age of 4, and regress over 10 years.

10 e – In adults the rule of 9's can be used, however in the paediatric population the proportionate body surface area depends on age. Half of 1 lower leg is 2.5%.

Chapter 9

Otolaryngology

Saba Ahmed

SAQs

1 Jack is a 6-year-old boy brought in by his mother to see you complaining of severe pain in his left ear.
  - **a** Give four further questions to ask when taking the history. (4 marks)
  - **b** From the history, you suspect a diagnosis of acute otitis media. Describe the appearance of his ear drum. (2 marks)
  - **c** Name two common organisms giving rise to this condition. (2 marks)
  - **d** State two complications of acute otitis media. (2 marks)
  - **e** Name two drugs you could prescribe in this case. (2 marks)

2 A concerned mother of a 3-year-old girl presents to you, her GP, with a 1-week history of lumps in the neck.
  - **a** What are the clinical features of tonsillitis? List four. (4 marks)
  - **b** Name two common causative organisms of tonsillitis. (2 marks)
  - **c** List two indications for tonsillectomy. (2 marks)
  - **d** Explain two aspects of your management plan for this patient. (2 marks)

3 Mrs Smith, a 44-year-old lady, has been referred to the outpatient clinic by her GP with a 5-week history of dizziness.
  - **a** Name three factors responsible for the maintenance of balance. (3 marks)
  - **b** Upon further questioning, you determine that the spells of dizziness last only for a very short duration, typically seconds to minutes when moving the head. What is your most likely diagnosis and how would you confirm the diagnosis clinically? (2 marks)
  - **c** Explain the pathophysiology of this condition. (2 marks)
  - **d** What is the treatment for the above condition? (1 mark)
  - **e** Describe the triad or symptoms commonly observed with Meniere's disease. (3 marks)
  - **f** Name one medical and one surgical treatment for Meniere's disease. (2 marks)

4 An 18-year-old male presents to A&E having sustained an injury to his nose whilst playing rugby.

- **a** Name two cartilaginous structures of the nose. (2 marks)
- **b** Give four further things you would ask about in the history. (4 marks)
- **c** Upon examination of the patient you discover the presence of a septal haematoma. What else would you look for on examination of this patient's nose? List two. (2 marks)
- **d** What complication can arise as a result of untreated septal haematoma? (1 mark)
- **e** What is the treatment of septal haematoma? (2 marks)

5 A 21-year-old gentleman presents to the local A&E with a nose bleed after being involved in a fight at a local pub.

- **a** Other than trauma, give four more causes of epistaxis. (4 marks)
- **b** State the name and location of the commonest site of bleeding. (2 marks)
- **c** As the first doctor to be reviewing this patient, after ABC what will form part of your initial assessment of this patient? (2 marks)
- **d** On examination of this patient you are able to visualise the bleeding point. Give three aspects of your management of his epistaxis? (3 marks)
- **e** The bleed is not alleviated by this procedure. What subsequent management options would you consider in this patient? Give two. (2 marks)

6 Mrs Kendrick, a 47-year-old lady, presents to you complaining of a hoarse voice.

- **a** Name the four cartilaginous structures that form the framework of the larynx. (4 marks)
- **b** Name the nerve supply to the intrinsic muscles of the larynx. (1 mark)
- **c** Give four further questions you would ask in the history. (4 marks)
- **d** Give two common causes of hoarseness of voice. (2 marks)
- **e** How may you visualise the vocal cords in clinic? (1 mark)

7 A 4-year-old boy presents to A&E with difficulty breathing. The mother gives a history that her son was playing with small toy cars when she noticed that he was struggling with his breathing. You suspect he has an inhaled foreign body.

- **a** Give two ways in which someone with an inhaled foreign body may present. (2 marks)
- **b** Name the imaging modality of choice to confirm or refute the diagnosis. (1 mark)

c Explain what is the most likely site of impaction in the airway for a foreign body and why. (2 marks)

d In some cases of respiratory obstruction a tracheostomy may be required. Describe the anatomical location for sighting a tracheostomy. (3 marks)

e Name four common complications of this procedure. (4 marks)

8 A 37-year-old female presents to her GP, complaining of a frontal headache, which is made worse on leaning forwards. A diagnosis of sinusitis is suspected.

a State four functions of the paranasal sinuses. (4 marks)

b Describe three clinical features of sinusitis, other than pain and headache. (3 marks)

c On viewing her medical records, you realise that this patient has previously presented with episodes of sinusitis in the past and you wish to investigate further in view of her recurrence. State two ways you could do this. (2 marks)

d Further investigation reveals no structural abnormality. Name two treatment options for this patient. (2 marks)

9 A 20-year-old female, who is currently 6 months pregnant presents to you with difficulty in hearing.

a How can deafness be classified? Give an example of each type. (4 marks)

b This patient is found to have otosclerosis. Describe this disease process. (2 marks)

c How might you clinically determine the type of deafness this patient is suffering from? (2 marks)

d What other symptoms might someone with a diagnosis of otosclerosis complain of, other than deafness? (2 marks)

e Give two treatment options for this patient. (2 marks)

10 A 27-year-old female presents to you complaining of a noticeable lump in the neck.

a Name two structures located in the anterior triangle of the neck. (2 marks)

b What further information would you like from the history? List four further aspects of history you should ask about. (4 marks)

c Examination findings reveal a cachexic female with irritability, diarrhoea and a central lump, woody in nature, which moves on swallowing, but not on protruding the tongue. Name the embryological remnant which results in a central neck lump which moves on protruding the tongue. (1 mark)

d From your findings you conclude a diagnosis of
Graves' disease. Name four possible findings on clinical
examination of this patient's eye. (4 marks)

e State three treatment options for hyperthyroidism. (3 marks)

EMQs

For each of the conditions listed below select the single most appropriate
presenting symptom from the list. Each answer may be used once, more than
once or not at all.

A Watery anterior rhinorrhoea, with post nasal drip
B Short-lived dizzy spells; seconds-minutes
C Ear pain with fever
D Discharge with itching and pain
E Dizzy spells lasting typically minutes to hours with tinnitus and deafness
F Nausea
G Weight loss

1 Acute otitis media.
2 BPPV.
3 Nasal polyps.
4 Meniere's disease.
5 Otitis externa.

For each of the conditions listed below select the most common causative
organism from the list. Each answer may be used once, more than once or
not at all.

A *Pseudomonas*
B *Pneumococcus*
C Non-infective cause
D *Haemophilus*
E Viral
F *Staphylococcus aureus*

6 Epiglottis.
7 Cholesteatoma.
8 Otitis externa.
9 Otitis media.
10 Laryngitis.

For each of the conditions listed below select the most useful investigation from the list. Each answer may be used once, more than once or not at all.

A Microlaryngoscopy
B Chest X-ray
C Endoscopic examination of nasal cavity
D Rinne's and Weber's test
E Audiogram
F Dix-Hallpike test

11 Nasal polyps.
12 Hoarse voice.
13 Otosclerosis.
14 Glue ear.
15 Benign paroxysmal positional vertigo (BPPV).

Match the treatment options with the conditions:
A Evacuation and application of pressure
B Surgery
C Reassurance as this condition usually resolves spontaneously
D Analgesia +/– amoxicillin
E Cyclizine for acute attacks.

16 Otitis media.
17 Meniere's disease.
18 Cholesteatoma.
19 Septal haematoma.
20 Glue ear.

Match the potential complications to the conditions:
A Cauliflower ear
B Mastoiditis and cerebellar abscess
C Retropharyngeal abscess and peritonsilar abscess
D Avascular necrosis
E Haemorrhage and damage to the oesophagus
F Facial paralysis and vertigo

21 Cholesteatoma.
22 Acute otitis media.
23 Septal haematoma.
24 Tracheostomy.
25 Tonsillitis.

MCQs

Please select one or more answers from the questions below.

1 Which of the following form part of the bony structure of the nose?
   a   Ethmoid bone
   b   Maxillary bone
   c   Zygoma
   d   Vomer
   e   Temporal bones
   f   Sphenoid bone

2 Which of the following statements are true for a patient diagnosed with left-sided glue ear, resulting in a conductive deafness?
   a   Rinne's negative on the left side, Weber's test sound lateralises to left side
   b   Rinne's positive on the left side, Weber's test sound lateralises to left side
   c   Rinne's positive on the left side, Weber's test central
   d   Rinne's negative on the left side, Weber's test sound lateralises to the right side
   e   Rinne's negative on the left side, Weber's test central

3 An audiogram for someone with presbyacusis shows:
   a   Low-frequency loss
   b   No changes from the normal picture
   c   High-frequency loss
   d   Uniform loss across all frequencies
   e   High- and low-frequency losses, with mid-range preserved

4 The single most common causative organism for otitis externa is:
   a   Fungal
   b   *Staph aureus*
   c   *Pseudomonas*
   d   *Lactobacillus*
   e   Viral

5 Cholesteatoma most commonly presents as:
   a   Conductive hearing loss
   b   Otalgia
   c   Facial palsy
   d   Offensive discharge
   e   Facial swelling

6   Clinical features of vestibular neuritis include:
   a   Vertigo
   b   Nystagmus
   c   Sensorineural deafness
   d   Conductive deafness
   e   Balance disturbances

7   Which of the following arteries do not form part of the anastomoses in Little's area?
   a   Anterior ethmoid artery
   b   Posterior ethmoid artery
   c   Greater palatine artery
   d   Lesser palatine artery
   e   Sphenopalatine artery
   f   Superior labial artery

8   Which of the following is the most likely diagnosis of a central neck lump, which moves on protruding the tongue?
   a   Branchial cyst
   b   Neck lipoma
   c   Lymphoma
   d   Thyroglossal cyst
   e   Pharyngeal pouch

9   The most common causative organism for acute epiglottitis is:
   a   *Staph. aureus*
   b   *Pseudomonas*
   c   *H. influenza*
   d   Viral
   e   *Strep. pneumoniae*

10   Which of the following are indications for tracheostomy:
   a   Prolonged intubation
   b   Airway obstruction
   c   Bronchial toilet
   d   Pleural effusion
   e   Septal haematoma of the nose

Answers

SAQs

1 **a** Fever
        Irritability
        Decreased oral intake
        Decreased urine output
        Vomiting
        Hearing impairment
        Recent upper respiratory tract infection (URTI)
        Duration of symptoms

    b Red
        Bulging ear drum
        Purulent discharge if perforated

    c *Streptococcus pneumoniae*
        Haemophilus influenza
        Moraxella catarrhalis
        Pseudomonas aeruginosa

    d Mastoiditis
        Cerebellar abscess
        Facial nerve palsy
        Meningitis
        Chronic otitis media

    e Analgesia such as paracetamol or ibuprofen.
        Antibiotics such as Amoxicillin. However, the benefits of antibiotics are arguable, as most cases are viral and therefore antibiotics only minimally improve the duration of disease or the symptoms.

Otitis media is inflammation of the middle ear from tympanic membrane to cochlea. Acute otitis media is usually viral. Otitis media with effusion occurs with eustachian tube dysfunction which causes negative pressure within the middle ear which, in turn, causes a collection of fluid within the middle ear and can affect hearing. If there is a bacterial infection within the middle ear and perforation occurs, this can lead to chronic suppurative otitis media. Treatment is usually symptomatic with analgesia and antipyretics but antibiotics may be required if there is a bacterial cause. Children who are suffering from chronic otitis media may require grommets inserting.

2   a   Sore throat
Halitosis
Pyrexia
Malaise
Difficulty swallowing
Fever
Lymphadenopathy
     b   Viral such as EBV, herpes simplex virus, CMV, adenovirus.
Group A beta-haemolytic streptococcus pyogenes.
Mycoplasma pneumoniae
     c   Chronic tonsillitis
Development of peritonsillar abscess (quinsy)
Suspected malignancy
Airway obstruction
Greater than six episodes of acute tonsillitis per year.
     d   Oral analgesia – paracetamol, NSAIDs, codeine
Topical analgesia – difflam
If very ill, or not improving, consider antibiotics such as penicillin
or erythromycin.
     f   Monospot test if suspected EBV

Tonsillitis is inflammation of the tonsils and may be viral or bacterial in origin, causing symptoms of sore throat, halitosis, swollen neck, otalgia, 'hot potato' voice and difficulty swallowing. Symptomatic treatment with paracetamol for fever and analgesia is the mainstay of treatment. If bacterial tonsillitis is suspected, a short course of penicillin V is effective. A common complication of tonsillitis is peritonsillar abscess (quinsy), which is more commonly seen in adults. Clinically, a displaced uvula may be seen as well as a history of odynophagia and drooling. Treatment for quinsy is incision and drainage under LA.

3   a   Vision
Proprioception
Labyrinthine activity
     b   BPPV
Dix-Hallpike test
     c   There is a phlebolith in the semicircular canal which continues
movement after the head has stopped moving, giving a transient
feeling of vertigo.
     d   Epley manoeuvre
     e   Episodic vertigo
Deafness
Tinnitus

f Medical (max. 1 mark) – betahistine, thiazide diuretics, prochlorperazine
Surgical (max. 1 mark) – grommet insertion, surgical labyrinthectomy

BPPV occurs when there is degenerative debris from the utricle floating freely in the semicircular canal causing symptoms of vertigo and nystagmus on head movements. Symptoms last 30–60 seconds. Meniere's disease is a triad of symptoms of vertigo, tinnitus and deafness caused by dilation of the endolymphatic spaces of the membranous labyrinth.

4 a Lateral nasal cartilage
Greater alar cartilage
Lesser alar cartilage
Nasal septum
b Epistaxis
Cerebrospinal fluid leakage
Loss of consciousness
Previous injuries
Time since injury
c Look for obvious deformity
Feel for steps in the contour
Extent of swelling
Lacerations
d Abscess of the nasal septum
Avascular necrosis of septal cartilage causing collapse of the nasal structure resulting in a deformity known as 'saddle nose'.
Perforation of the nasal septum.
e Evacuation under GA with suture and packing to prevent re-accumulation.

Nasal trauma can lead to a septal haematoma – this is a blood-filled cavity between the cartilage and supporting perichondrium. As cartilage is dependent on the perichondrium for its blood supply it is important for the haematoma to be drained urgently and packed as this prevents avascular necrosis.

5 a Idiopathic
Local infection
Inflammatory
Iatrogenic
Anticoagulants
Coagulopathies
Neoplasm

   b   Little's area
       Found on the nasal septum
   c   Is there active bleeding?
       Assess for signs of shock – pale, tachycardia, hypotensive
   d   Firm constant pressure on nostrils for 10 minutes.
       Topical adrenaline
       Nasal cautery
   e   Anterior nasal pack
       Posterior nasal pack
       Surgical interventions – rigid nasendoscopy and electrocautery, artery ligations, embolisation of vessels under radiographic control.

Ninety percent of epistaxis is from Little's area which is in the anteroinferior part of the nasal septum and is also known as Kiesselbach's plexus. This is a highly vascular area of the nose and it is important to both stop the bleeding and then treat the underlying cause.

6 **a**   Epiglottis
       Thyroid cartilage
       Cricoid cartilage
       Arytenoid cartilage
   b   Recurrent laryngeal nerve
   c   Duration
       Preceding infection
       Associated acid reflux
       Chest problems
       Smoking
       Alcohol
       Weight loss
   d   Laryngopharyngeal reflux
       Laryngitis
       Reinke's oedema
       Vocal cord nodules
       Laryngeal nerve palsy
   e   Flexible nasal endoscopy

Laryngopharyngeal reflux occurs with chronic GORD and as such medical treatment with PPIs or surgical fundoplication can benefit patients. Reinke's oedema is a gelatinous fusiform enlargement of the vocal cords due to chronic cord irritation which is commonest in middle aged females and smokers.

7 a Persistent monophonic wheeze
Pyrexia with productive cough secondary to pulmonary suppuration
Asymptomatic
Recurrent chest infections
  b Chest X-ray
  c Right main bronchus
Wider calibre and straighter path than the left main bronchus.
  d In the midline directly below the level of the thyroid cartilage through the cricothyroid membrane.
  e Intra-operative – haemorrhage, damage to trachea, injury to paratracheal structures
Early post-operative – haemorrhage, infection, swallowing difficulty
Late – tracheal stenosis, tracheocutaneous or tracheo-oesophageal fistula
Blocking of tracheostomy

A tracheostomy may be performed electively or as an emergency procedure if the airway if irreversibly compromised. The tracheostomy is created immediately below the level of the thyroid cartilage by making a hole through the cricothyroid membrane.

8 a Decrease the weight of the cranium
Humidify inspired air
Warm inspired air
Resonance chamber for inspired air
Provide a buffer against facial trauma
Insulation for sensitive facial structures
  b Nasal discharge
Anosmia
Fever
Lethargy
  c Rigid nasal endoscopy
CT scan
  d Analgesia
Antibiotics
Nasal decongestants
Functional endoscopic sinus surgery (FESS)

FESS unblocks sinuses and promotes better natural drainage. This can be performed for people with persistent or severe sinus infections and nasal polyps.

9   a   Conductive deafness – perforated tympanic membrane, external canal obstruction, eustachian tube dysfunction
Sensorineural deafness – trauma, Meniere's disease, ototoxic drugs

b   Vascular spongy bone replaces the normal lamellar bone of the otic capsule.

c   Rinne's test in combination with Weber's test.

d   Tinnitus

e   Hearing aid
Cochlear implant
Stapedectomy

Otosclerosis is an autosomal dominant condition in which there is abnormal growth of the middle ear bones leading to a progressive conductive deafness. Otosclerosis presents in early adult life.

10   a   Carotid sheath
Thyroid gland
Parathyroid glands
Submandibular gland

b   About the lump – duration, position, pain
Associated symptoms – dysphonia, otalgia, fever
Smoking
Alcohol

c   Thyroglossal cyst

d   Exophthalmos
Lid retraction
Lid lag
Ophthalmoplegia
Chemosis

e   Antithyroid drugs e.g. carbimazole, propylthiouracil
Radio-iodine
Surgery

Graves' disease is the commonest cause of hyperthyroidism. It is commoner in women than men. It is an auto-immune disease in which serum IgG antibodies bind to and activate the TSH receptor resulting in the production of thyroid hormone.

EMQs

1   **C**
2   **B**
3   **A** – Nasal polyps also present with nasal obstruction and changes in voice quality
4   **E**
5   **D**
6   **D**
7   **C**
8   **A** – *Pseudomonas* is the commonest organism, *staphylococcus aureus* is another common causative organism
9   **B**
10 **E** – Mainly viral in nature but can also be due to GORD or infections with *strep* or *staph* species
11 **C**
12 **A**
13 **D** – Reveals a sensorineural loss
14 **E** – May also conduct impedance audiometry to help distinguish glue ear from simple eustachian tube dysfunction
15 **F** – This condition is assessed clinically, a positive Dix-Hallpike test is indicated by rotational nystagmus
16 **D**
17 **E**
18 **B**
19 **A**
20 **C** – Reassurance with 3 monthly follow-up, if it does not resolve then could treat with antibiotics and steroid ear drops
21 **F**
22 **B** – Acute otitis media can also lead to complications of facial palsy and meningitis
23 **D**
24 **E**
25 **C**

MCQs

1 a and d – The structure of the nose is comprised of both cartilage and bone.

2 a – Rinne's compares air conduction with bone conduction. Normally air conduction is loudest (Rinne's positive) but if the findings are reversed this is suggestive of conductive deafness.

Weber's test is performed by placing a tuning fork on the patient's forehead and asking which side the sound localises to. Normally there is no localisation of sound. In conductive deafness sound will localise to the affected side and in sensorineural deafness sound will lateralise away from the affected side.

3 c – Presbyacusis is hearing impairment due to the progressive degeneration of hearing in the auditory system. Audiograms demonstrate high frequency hearing loss.

4 c – Otitis externa is inflammation of the outer ear and canal and is also known as 'swimmer's ear'. It is usually due to a bacterial infection and symptoms include otalgia, itching and a watery discharge. The treatment options include aural toilet, and topical antibiotics.

5 d – A cholesteatoma occurs when there is growth of keratinised squamous epithelium in the middle ear. This is locally destructive to surrounding structures and leads to a foul smelling discharge, deafness, headache and may lead to facial paralysis.

6 a and d – Vestibular neuritis is the inflammation of the vestibular nerve and ganglion usually due to a viral URTI. Symptoms are usually unilateral but may include vertigo, nystagmus and vomiting. Prochlorperazine (a vestibular sedative) may be helpful for patients.

7 b and d – Little's area, located in the anteroinferior part of the nasal septum, also known as Kiesselbach's plexus is a highly vascular area of the nasal septum due to the anastomosis of four vessels.

8 d – A thyroglossal cyst is a remnant of the thyroglossal duct. During development the thyroid gland descends from the foramen caecum to its final adult anatomical position. The thyroglossal duct is formed at its descent and normally obliterates during development but if any part of the tract persists it can give rise to a fistula, sinus or cyst.

9 c – Epiglottis is most often seen in 3–7 year olds. It is a life-threatening medical condition and it is vital that examination is not attempted in case the airway becomes compromised. The child will have obvious respiratory distress and dysphagia and be drooling.

10 a and b and c – Tracheostomy may be performed in the emergency setting, or due to impaired respiratory function, to assist weaning, or to help clear airway secretions.

Chapter 10

Plastic surgery

Philip Stather

SAQs

1 An 18-year-old gentleman attends A&E having trapped his left fingers in a gate. He has a subungal haematoma on his index finger, a laceration to his middle finger nailbed, and his ring finger nail is hanging off.

    a How does a nail grow? (1 mark)

    b What vaccine must you ensure is up-to-date in this gentleman? (1 mark)

    c How can you treat a subungal haematoma? (1 mark)

    d This gentleman has an extremely tender middle and ring finger, and you therefore arrange an X-ray of these digits. This reveals a fracture of the distal phalanx of the middle finger. What type of fracture is this and what further medication is required for this patient? (2 marks)

    e What treatment is required for the ring finger, and what advice should the patient be given regarding the nail? (2 marks)

    f The middle finger is treated by excision of the nail followed by suturing the wound and replacement of the nail. What further treatment is required regarding the fracture? (1 mark)

    g Another patient comes in with an infection around the nail bed. What is this called? (1 mark)

    h If left untreated, how may this spread? (2 marks)

2 A 30-year-old gentleman weighing 70 kg is admitted following spilling boiling water down the front of his left leg.

    a Give two causes of burns other than thermal. (2 marks)

    b What percentage burns does this patient have? (1 mark)

    c Calculate his fluid requirements over the next 24 hours, and explain how this should be divided. (2 marks)

    d Give three reasons for admission to a specialist burns centre. (3 marks)

    e List three features of a full thickness burn. (3 marks)

    f Apart from calculating the percentage burn and starting fluid, give two other aspects of management for this patient. (2 marks)

g   In circumferential burns what further procedure may be
    required?   (1 mark)

3   A young gentleman has been treated for third degree burns to his left
    thigh. Following debridement of necrotic tissue, it is determined that he
    requires a skin graft.
    a   Name the two types of skin graft used.   (2 marks)
    b   Give two advantages of using a skin graft.   (2 marks)
    c   What can be done to increase the size of the graft,
        which also prevents fluid collecting underneath the graft? (1 mark)
    d   Give three complications you should warn the patient
        about.   (3 marks)
    e   Explain the differences between a skin graft and a flap. (2 marks)

4   A 60-year-old gentleman has come to see you regarding a growth on his
    shin. It is black and you suspect a malignant melanoma.
    a   Give three local signs or symptoms you will ask about to
        aid your diagnosis.   (3 marks)
    b   How can you establish a definitive diagnosis in this case? (1 mark)
    c   Give two common areas for metastases to occur.   (2 marks)
    d   Name one staging system for malignant melanomas. (1 mark)
    e   For how long should this patient be followed up, and
        what two areas should you examine during follow up visits? (3 marks)

5   A 70-year-old gentleman comes to see you regarding multiple lesions on
    his forehead which have appeared over the past year.
    a   Rank the types of skin cancer from most to least likely
        to metastasise.   (3 marks)
    b   Give three risk factors for developing skin cancer. (3 marks)
    c   List three strategies you would advise patients to take to
        prevent skin cancer developing.   (3 marks)
    d   Give two non-surgical treatment options for a rodent
        ulcer.   (2 marks)

6   Amy, a 22-year-old girl comes to see you in clinic regarding breast
    reduction surgery.
    a   Give the medical term for this procedure.   (1 mark)
    b   This type of surgery is not usually available on the
        NHS. What three aspects of this patient's history must
        be assessed in order to determine suitability?   (3 marks)
    c   Give three symptoms this patient may suffer with. (3 marks)
    d   You are asked to take consent from the patient. Give
        four complications specific to this procedure which you
        will seek her consent for.   (4 marks)

7 A 25-year-old lady comes to see you in your private clinic regarding breast implants.

   a Give three indications for breast augmentation. (3 marks)
   b Name the two types of implants used for this procedure. (2 marks)
   c Give three specific complications of breast augmentation. (3 marks)
   d What is the typical life expectancy of an implant? (1 mark)
   e Name one type of incision which can be used in the procedure. (1 mark)

8 A 35-year-old black woman comes to see you regarding a large 'ugly' scar which has appeared following a caesarean section. Whilst in clinic, she also mentions that she has noticed some thickening of the skin on her hand.

   a What is the name for this type of scarring? (1 mark)
   b What is the cause of this type of scarring? (1 mark)
   c Give two options for preventing this condition. (2 marks)
   d She opts for surgical excision of the scar. What is the recurrence rate for this condition? (1 mark)
   e You examine her hand and notice a thickening of the palmar aponeurosis over the 4th digit. What is this condition? (1 mark)
   f You decide to assess her hand function. Give three common activities you would ask about. (3 marks)
   g You refer her for surgical intervention. Given the potential of keloid scarring with open surgery, give two alternative interventions that could be used. (2 marks)

9 A 45-year-old man is caught in a house fire, and escapes with burns to his chest, face and hands.

   a Give two signs and two symptoms of inhalation injury. (4 marks)
   b His oxygen saturations are 99% on air on examination, however, his respiratory rate is 25 and his blood gas shows a pO_2 of only 8. Please explain these results. (2 marks)
   c What two treatments can you give to improve his breathing? (2 marks)
   d On further examination of his chest, you noticed that the scars are circumferential. Why may this cause breathing difficulties, and what treatment may be required? (2 marks)

10 A 28-year-old man comes to see you regarding his weight. He currently weighs 120 kg and is 1.7 metres tall.

    a   Calculate his BMI. (1 mark)

    b   He is complaining of a rash underneath his breasts. What is the name for male breast enlargement? (1 mark)

    c   Suggest the most common type of causative organism for his rash. (1 mark)

    d   Give one type of cream which may help with his rash. (1 mark)

    e   He has tried numerous methods of weight loss, and asks for referral for gastric banding. Give two groups of patients who may be eligible for gastric band surgery. (2 marks)

    f   Give two possible complications of gastric band surgery. (2 marks)

    g   Post-surgery the patient has a good result with significant weight loss, however, he is left with considerable amounts of excess skin. What is the name for the surgical removal of this? (1 mark)

    h   After initial good results your patient attends complaining his weight loss has stopped. What could be done to further increase his weight loss? (1 mark)

EMQs

Calculate the initial rate of fluid per hour for these burns patients:

A   100 ml
B   125 ml
C   300 ml
D   375 ml
E   400 ml
F   500 ml
G   750 ml
H   1000 ml

1   80 kg man with 15% burns.
2   70 kg woman with 20% burns arriving 1 hour after injury.
3   50 kg woman with 10% burns.
4   100 kg man with 15% burns.
5   90 kg man with 25% burns arriving 2 hours after injury.

Match the description with the diagnosis:
A Malignant melanoma
B Neurofibroma
C Kaposi's sarcoma
D Squamous cell carcinoma
E Strawberry naevus
F Bowen's disease
G Basal cell carcinoma

6 An ulcerated rapidly spreading lesion with everted edges.
7 Patient with multiple small subcutaneous lumps. You notice café-au-lait spots.
8 A premalignant condition causing a raised red, hyperkeratotic lesion.
9 A pearly white lesion with a rolled edge.
10 A red raised compressible lesion in a 2-week-old baby.

Calculate the percentage of surface area burns.
A 1%
B 4.5%
C 9%
D 18%
E 20%
F 27%
G 37%

11 An 18-year-old man has spilt boiling water on his left lower leg.
12 A 60-year-old man who has obtained an electrical burn to his right hand.
13 An 18-year-old man who fell into a chemical vat from the waist up.
14 A 20-year-old girl with severe sunburn to her entire back.
15 A 70-year-old lady burnt herself with an iron on the back of her arm.

Match the disease to the description:
A Basal cell carcinoma
B Squamous cell carcinoma
C Malignant melanoma
D Kaposi sarcoma
E Bowen's disease
F Keratoacanthoma

16 A pigmented lesion which has been bleeding and itching.
17 A premalignant condition presenting as a well-demarcated erythematous plaque.
18 A small lesion with a pearly white appearance.

19 A rapidly growing red ulcer.
20 A rapidly growing lesion which regresses spontaneously.

Match the suture with the description:
A Prolene
B Onocryl
C Vicryl Rapide
D Vicryl
E Ethilon
F Silk
G Steel

21 Multifilament material lasting roughly a week.
22 Non-absorbable material often used for suturing drains.
23 Monofilament absorbable suture used in skin closure.
24 Used for closure of median sternotomy.
25 A synthetic monofilament non-absorbable suture.

MCQs

1 A 60 kg woman is admitted 2 hours after sustaining 10% burns. What is her initial hourly fluid rate?
  a   2400 ml
  b   300 ml
  c   400 ml
  d   200 ml
  e   1200 ml

2 An allogeneic graft is:
  a   From a different site on the same individual's body
  b   A synthetic material
  c   A graft from a different species
  d   A graft from a twin
  e   A graft from the same species

3 What is the appropriate excision margin for a malignant melanoma with a Breslow depth of 1.5 mm?
  a   Clear margins
  b   1 cm
  c   1–2 cm
  d   2 cm
  e   2–3 cm

4   What is the 5-year survival for a patient with a malignant melanoma with a Breslow thickness of 3 mm?
    a   100%
    b   95–100%
    c   80–95%
    d   60–75%
    e   50%

5   Which of these skin conditions is malignant?
    a   Bowen's disease
    b   Keratoacanthoma
    c   Papilloma
    d   Lipoma
    e   Neurofibroma

6   A 16-year-old boy comes to A&E with a subungal haematoma. What is the most appropriate treatment for this condition?
    a   Excision of the nail
    b   Trephination
    c   No treatment
    d   Neighbour strapping
    e   X-ray

7   Risk factors for skin flap failure include:
    a   Smoking
    b   Hypertension
    c   Haematoma formation
    d   Infection
    e   All of the above

8   Which of the following is not a complication of breast augmentation surgery?
    a   Infection
    b   Haematoma
    c   Areola denervation
    d   Implant rupture
    e   Nipple discharge

9 Which statement is false regarding breast reduction surgery?
  a Breast reduction is always free on the NHS
  b Breast reduction surgery may damage the innervation to the nipple
  c Breast reduction may cause difficulty with breastfeeding
  d Back pain is a common reason for patients wanting breast reduction surgery
  e Patient may have a recurrence of their symptoms through weight gain

10 Which statement is untrue regarding Botox injections?
  a They block noradrenaline receptors
  b Block acetylcholine release at the pre-synaptic membrane
  c Botox can be injected into muscular contractures for symptomatic relief
  d Botox can be injected into the anal sphincter to treat anal fissure
  e The effects of botox last on average 4 months

Answers

SAQs

1 a   From the nail bed
  b   Tetanus
  c   Trephining the nail (drilling a hole through the nail into the haematoma)
  d   Open or compound fracture
      Will require antibiotics
  e   Removal of the nail which may be re-implanted to keep the wound covered.
      Advised that if there is damage to the nail bed then the nail may not regrow as previously.
  f   Neighbour strapping
  g   Paronychia
  h   This may cause cellulitis, which may spread to the deep space and flexor tendon sheaths.

Nails grow from the growth plate in the nail bed at a rate of 0.1 mm per day. Injuries require prompt treatment to prevent further damage and ensure a good cosmetic result, however if damage occurs to the nail bed the nail may not grow as it previously did.

2 a   Chemical
      Electrical
      Radiation
  b   9%
  c $4 \times 70 \times 9 = 2520$ ml Hartmann's
      1260 ml over first 8 hours, then 1260 ml over following 16 hours
  d   Burns to the face, eyes, ears, hands, feet, genitalia, perineum, and over joints.
      Burns greater than 10% in children or 20% in adults.
      Full thickness burns greater than 5%.
      Burns in patients with significant comorbidities or trauma
      Inhalation injury.
      Significant electrical or chemical burns.
  e   Leathery
      Skin appears waxy white
      Painless dry surface
      Does not blanch

f   Analgesia
    Wound care
    Tetanus
g   Escharotomy

The rule of 9's is used to determine the percentage body surface area burned; with 9% each for the head and arms, and 9% each for the front and back of the legs, 18% for the front of the torso and 18% for the back of the torso, with 1% for the genitals.

Parklands formula states that 4 ml/kg/% body surface area burned should be given over the next 24 hours, with half over the first 8 hours, and half over the following 16 hours, starting at the time of the burn, not the time of admission.

3 a   Full thickness
           Partial thickness
       b   Cosmetic appearance
           Faster healing
           Reduced hospital stay
       c   The graft is meshed
       d   Bleeding
           Infection
           Loss of grafted skin
           Nerve damage
           Pain from the donor site
           Cosmesis
       e   A skin flap retains its own blood supply and is used in areas
           requiring better cosmesis, or when covering specialised tissue such
           as gliding tendons. Skin grafts are transplanted material from one
           part of the body to another. They are frequently meshed to increase
           the area they may cover. They initially gain nutrition directly from
           plasma in the base of the wound until angiogenesis occurs after
           roughly 36 hours. Good wound care is required on the donor and
           recipient site to prevent wound infections.

Skin grafts are often used to treat burns, and wounds which are too large to heal naturally, such as post-necrotising fasciitis excision, or with large skin tumours. They may be full thickness or partial thickness, and are often meshed to increase the surface area they may cover.

4 a Change in size
Change in shape
Change in colour
Diameter > 7 mm
Inflammation
Crusting or bleeding
Satellite lesions

   b Excision biopsy

   c Liver
Bone
Brain
Lungs
GIT

   d Breslow thickness – the depth of invasion of the tumour
Clark's level – the anatomical invasion of the tumour into the dermis

   e 5 years
Excision site for local recurrence
All lymph nodes

Malignant melanomas are often brown or black pigmented irregular lesions which commonly occur on the lower limbs, feet, head and neck. Signs of malignancy include new lesions, an increase in size, colour or pigmentation, bleeding, crusting, ulceration, pain, satellite lesions, and lymphadenopathy. They should be excised with a wide margin depending on the Breslow thickness.

5 a Malignant melanoma
Squamous cell carcinoma
Basal cell carcinoma

   b Sunlight exposure
Radiation exposure
Chemical carcinogens such as coal and arsenic
Genetics
Chronic ulceration

   c Wear a hat and sunglasses
Use sunblock with a high protection factor
Stay out of the sun between 11 and 3 o'clock

   d Cryotherapy
Radiotherapy
Medical therapy in the form of aldara or imiquomod cream for superficial spreading types.

Skin cancer is increasing due to the increased number of foreign holidays and use of sun beds. Basal cell carcinomas typically occur on the nose, and have a raised rolled pearly edge with superficial dilated blood vessels over the surface. They may be locally invasive but metastasise rarely. Squamous cell carcinomas can spread rapidly locally, and occasionally metastasise to regional lymph nodes. It is typically an ulcerated lesion with everted edges.

6 a Reduction mammoplasty
   b Biological – back pain
      Psychological
      Social
   c Back pain
      Neck pain
      Skin irritation
      Difficulty playing sport
      Psychological distress
   d Difficulty breastfeeding
      Asymmetry
      Altered nipple sensation
      Fluid retention in the breast
      Altered erogenous function
      Recurrence

Breast reduction surgery is not funded on the NHS routinely as it is cosmetic surgery. Patients must prove that they have significant pain, psychological and social problems from this, and their GP should refer the case to the PCT for consideration of funding.

7 a Primary reconstruction following mastectomy.
      Revision reconstruction to improve the result of a previous reconstruction.
      Primary augmentation for cosmetic reasons.
      Revision reconstruction to improve the result of a previous augmentation.
      Sex change operations.
   b Saline
      Silicone
   c Capsular contracture
      Rupture
      Infection
      Poor cosmesis
      Mastectomy

    d   10–15 years, although this is improving

    e   Inframammary fold

        Periareolar

        Axillary

Breast augmentation is the most common form of cosmetic surgery, typically in young women, sex change operations, or following mastectomy.

8 **a**   Keloid scar

    b   An overgrowth of granulation tissue at the site of injury.

    c   Avoid abrasions

        Avoid injury

        Avoid unnecessary surgery

    d   Over 50%

    e   Dupuytren's contracture

    f   Fastening buttons

        Using cutlery

        Dressing

        Washing

        Grip a page

        Hold a pen

        Opposition

        Grip

    g   Collagenase injection – the cords are dissolved by the injection of collagenase

        Needle aponeuorotomy – weakening the cords through insertion and manipulation of a needle

Keloid scars are more common in the black population, due to abrasions or operative scars. Treatment is usually through prevention, by avoiding injuries, and avoiding unessential surgery.

9 **a**   Signs – burns to the nose mouth and face, singed nostril hairs, carbonaceous sputum

        Symptoms – coughing, vomiting, nausea, sleepiness, confusion

    b   He has increased levels of carboxyhaemoglobin in the blood.

        On pulse oximetry this shows the same as oxyhaemoglobin so gives a falsely high reading.

    c   High flow oxygen

        Bronchodilators

    d   Decreases chest expansion

        Escharotomy

Inhalation injury is the most common cause for death in patients following burns. Patients require high flow oxygen and bronchodilators, and often require intubation in severe cases.

10 a $120/(1.7 \times 1.7) = 41.5$
   b Gynaecomastia
   c Fungal
   d Clotrimazole
      Miconazole
      Terbinafine
      Any other antifungal cream
   e BMI > 40
      BMI 35–40 with comorbidities known to improve with weight loss
   f Productive burping
      Ulceration
      Gastritis
      Erosion
      Slippage of band
      Port site pain
      Nausea and vomiting
      Diarrhoea
      Infection of band or port site
      Band over or under inflation
   g Apronectomy
   h Tighten the band

Obesity is a major health problem, with an increasing number of patients undergoing bariatric surgery. It is important to know which patients are eligible for gastric banding, and how to advise them regarding weight loss and post-operative complications.

EMQs

1	**C**	10	**E**	19	**B**
2	**E**	11	**B**	20	**F**
3	**B**	12	**A**	21	**C**
4	**D**	13	**G**	22	**F**
5	**G**	14	**D**	23	**B**
6	**D**	15	**A**	24	**G**
7	**B**	16	**C**	25	**A**
8	**F**	17	**E**		
9	**G**	18	**A**		

MCQs

1 d – Parklands formula is 4 × kg × % burns = 4 × 60 × 10 = 2400 ml over 24 hours. Half of this given over the first 8 hours is 1200 ml. She has arrived after 2 hours, therefore 1200 ml over 6 hours is 200 ml per hour.

2 e – An autologous graft is from a different site on the same individual's body. An isogeneic graft is from a twin. An allogeneic graft is from the same species. A xenogeneic graft is from a different species. A prosthetic is artificial.

3 c – A melanoma *in situ* requires clear margin excision. Breslow thickness < 1 mm requires a 1 cm excision margin. Breslow thickness 1–2 mm requires a 1–2 cm margin. Breslow thickness 2.1–4 mm requires a margin of 2 cm. Breslow thickness >4 mm requires a 2–3 cm margin.

4 d – A melanoma *in situ* has a 100% 5 year survival. Breslow thickness <1 mm has a 95–100% 5 year survival. Breslow thickness 1–2 mm has an 80–95% 5 year survival. Breslow thickness 2.1–4 mm has a 60–75% 5 year survival. Breslow thickness >4 mm has a 50% 5 year survival.

5 a – Bowen's disease is a premalignant skin change producing a raised red hyperkeratotic lesion. It can be treated with 5-fluorouracil, cryotherapy or surgical excision.

6 b – Trephining the nail involves drilling a hold through the nail to evacuate the haematoma, which restores the blood supply in the area.

7 e – There are pre-operative causes of skin flap failure such as poor design, inadequate size, or traumatised tissue, intra-operative causes such as too much tension, damage to the blood supply or kinking the pedicle, post-operative causes such as haematoma formation and infection, and patient factors such as smoking and hypertension.

8 e – Nipple discharge is not a complication of breast augmentation surgery.

9 a – Breast reduction surgery is only funded on the NHS after funding applications and assessment of the patient from a biopsychosocial perspective.

10 a – Botulinum toxin works by blocking the release of acetylcholine at the pre-synaptic membrane. It has several potential uses as described above, as well as in the removal of facial lines.

Chapter 11

Cardiothoracic surgery

Philip Stather

SAQs

1 A 30-year-old lady is admitted after being kicked in the chest by a horse. She has severe pain over her right lower ribs.
  - **a** Which ribs are true ribs, false ribs, and floating ribs? (3 marks)
  - **b** You perform a chest X-ray which shows a flail chest. What is the definition of a flail chest? (2 marks)
  - **c** How can you assess clinically for a flail segment? (1 mark)
  - **d** Her chest X-ray reveals no underlying lung injuries, and her observations are stable. Give three aspects of her management in this case. (3 marks)
  - **e** If the flail segment was to cause a bruise to the underlying lung, what would be the name of this condition? (1 mark)

2 A 20-year-old man is brought into A&E resus following a high speed car crash.
  - **a** According to ATLS guidelines what are the first two aspects of his management you should ensure? (2 marks)
  - **b** While assessing him you notice he has a very rapid respiratory rate, and his oxygen saturations are 80%. You suspect he may have a tension pneumothorax. Give four signs you would expect on clinical examination. (4 marks)
  - **c** What immediate management will you initiate? (2 marks)
  - **d** Following this procedure his breathing improves somewhat. Regarding his chest what further management is required? (2 marks)

3 A 25-year-old girl was a passenger in a car crash. The driver died on impact, however, she has been brought in on a spinal board with oxygen and fluids running, and is maintaining her own airway.

    a On primary survey you notice that her respiratory rate is 30 and oxygen saturations 85%. Give four other aspects of examination you will do to determine the cause of her respiratory distress. (4 marks)

    b You suspect a haemothorax. What percentage of a patient's blood volume can be lost in the pleural space? (1 mark)

    c What may you see on chest X-ray to indicate haemothorax? (1 mark)

    d You decide to insert a chest drain. Where in relation to the rib should you insert the chest drain and why? (2 marks)

    e Give two indications for emergency thoracotomy in patients with haemothorax. (2 marks)

4 A 60-year-old man presents to A&E due to a tearing pain in his chest. You suspect he has an aortic dissection.

    a Give three other symptoms of aortic dissection. (3 marks)

    b Give three causes of aortic dissection. (3 marks)

    c What characteristic signs may you see on chest X-ray? (1 mark)

    d What is the mortality rate for this condition? (1 mark)

    e Give two reasons why this patient may develop a pleural effusion. (2 marks)

5 A 14-year-old boy is brought to see you in clinic complaining that his chest is an odd shape. He feels that he has a sunken sternum and ribs.

    a What is the term for a sunken sternum and ribs? (1 mark)

    b What is the term for a protrusion of the sternum and ribs? (1 mark)

    c Give one common syndrome associated with this boy's condition. (1 mark)

    d Explain why this condition is more evident in males. (1 mark)

    e Give one non-surgical treatment option for this patient. (1 mark)

    f How is this condition corrected surgically? (1 mark)

    g Give three complications of this surgery. (3 marks)

6 A 62-year-old lady comes to see you regarding repeated episodes of collapse. On examination, you find an ejection systolic murmur radiating to the carotids.

    a What is the most likely diagnosis in this patient? (1 mark)

    b Give three common symptoms the patient may suffer from other than collapse. (3 marks)

    c Suggest two possible causes of this condition. (2 marks)

d   Following thorough investigation it is decided that a
valve replacement is required. Give the two different
types of valve that can be used, and one advantage and
disadvantage of each.   (4 marks)

7   A young boy is seen regarding recurrent cyanotic spells. He is diagnosed
with tetralogy of Fallot.
a   List two further causes of congenital cardiac cyanosis.   (2 marks)
b   What are the four abnormalities present in tetralogy of
Fallot?   (4 marks)
c   Other than cyanosis, give three symptoms of tetralogy
of Fallot.   (3 marks)
d   *In utero*, there is a communication between the left and
right atria which closes at birth. What is the name of this? (1 mark)

8   A 64-year-old gentleman comes to see you in clinic due to recurrent
episodes of chest pain. This comes on during walking, and he must stop
whilst climbing the stairs.
a   What is the term for this condition?   (1 mark)
b   Give three risk factors for this disease.   (3 marks)
c   At what stage during the cardiac cycle do the coronary
arteries receive their blood supply?   (1 mark)
d   Despite optimising his medical management his pain
persists. Give two further interventions which may help
this patient.   (2 marks)
e   What imaging will you require to determine which of
your above treatments is most appropriate?   (1 mark)
f   You decide to refer the patient to the cardiothoracic
surgeons for surgical intervention. Name two possible
vessels that may be used for grafting.   (2 marks)

9   You are referred a newborn baby with a patent ductus arteriosus (PDA).
a   Where does the ductus arteriosus connect?   (1 mark)
b   Give three symptoms of a PDA.   (3 marks)
c   Give three signs of a PDA.   (3 marks)
d   What imaging modality is used to diagnose a PDA?   (1 mark)
e   Give three methods of closing a PDA.   (3 marks)

10 You are referred a 70-year-old otherwise healthy man who has a suspicious lesion on his chest X-ray, and symptoms of a pancoast tumour.

    a List three symptoms differentiating a pancoast tumour from lung cancer. (3 marks)

    b Give three risk factors for developing lung cancer. (3 marks)

    c What is the most common treatment for this condition? (1 mark)

    d How many lobes does the left lung contain? (1 mark)

    e How many segments does the right lung contain, and why is this knowledge relevant? (2 marks)

11 A 40-year-old man is admitted following a head-on collision at 50 mph. On examination, you suspect he has a cardiac tamponade.

    a Give three signs of cardiac tamponade. (3 marks)

    b What may be seen on this patient's chest X-ray? (1 mark)

    c Give one further investigation that can be done in A&E to diagnose this condition. (1 mark)

    d Whilst you are assessing this patient his heart goes into a shockable rhythm. Give two shockable heart rhythms. (2 marks)

    e You manage to resuscitate him successfully, and need to treat his cardiac tamponade. Name and explain the emergency treatment of this condition. (3 marks)

EMQs

Match these post-operative complications with the description below:

A Cardiac tamponade
B PE
C DVT
D MI
E Pleural effusion
F Haemothorax
G Pneumothorax

1 Post chest drain removal a patient becomes increasingly short of breath, with decreased chest expansion and resonance to percussion.

2 A patient post coronary artery bypass graft (CABG) pulls out his pericardial drains. Over the next few hours his blood pressure drops, and JVP rises.

3 A patient 3-days post-op becomes acutely short of breath with chest pain. You perform an ECG which shows q waves and t waves in lead III.

4 A patient 2-days post-op has chest pain and shortness of breath. You perform an ECG which shows a new left bundle branch block.

5 A gentleman has difficulty mobilising post-mitral valve repair. He develops pain in his left calf, which is made worse on passive flexion.

Match the blood pressure with the anatomical location.
A 2–6 mmHg
B 15–25 mmHg
C 8–15 mmHg
D 60–90 mmHg
E 90–140 mmHg

6 Arterial systolic blood pressure.
7 Right atrial pressure.
8 Right ventricular diastolic pressure.
9 Arterial diastolic blood pressure.
10 Right ventricular systolic pressure.

Match the following clinical signs and diagnosis:
A Pneumothorax
B Tension pneumothorax
C Haemothorax
D Cardiac tamponade
E Pneumonia
F Chronic obstructive pulmonary disease

11 Decreased chest expansion, dullness to percussion, decreased breath sounds.
12 Raised JVP, muffled heart sounds.
13 Left-sided hyper-resonance to percussion, no breath sounds.
14 Dull left base to percussion, coarse crepitations.
15 Decreased breath sounds, decreased vocal resonance, resonance to percussion.

Match the following clinical signs and diagnosis:
A Aortic stenosis
B Aortic sclerosis
C Aortic regurgitation
D Mitral stenosis
E Mitral regurgitation
F Pulmonary stenosis
G Tricuspid regurgitation
H PDA
I Endocarditis

16 A systolic murmur radiating to the carotids.
17 A pansystolic murmur radiating to the axilla.
18 A bounding JVP, with a systolic murmur.
19 A continuous machinery murmur.
20 Early diastolic murmur.

Match the following lung function tests with the description below:
A Peak expiratory flow rate
B Forced vital capacity
C Functional residual capacity
D Forced expiratory volume
E Residual volume
F Forced expiratory volume
G Total lung capacity

21 The volume of air in the lungs following a normal exhaled breath.
22 A measure of how quickly you can exhale.
23 The volume of air exhaled forcibly in a single breath, typically over 1 second.
24 The volume of air in the lungs after full inspiration.
25 The volume of air in the lungs following forced expiration.

MCQs

1 Where should you place a cannula to decompress a tension pneumothorax?
  a Mid-axillary line 2nd intercostal space
  b Anterior axillary line 5th intercostal space
  c Anterior axillary line 2nd intercostal space
  d Mid-clavicular line 4th intercostal space
  e Mid-clavicular line 2nd intercostal space

2 What is the most common cardiac abnormality in patients with Down syndrome?
  a Ventriculo septal defect (VSD)
  b Atrioventricular septal defect (AVSD)
  c Tetralogy of Fallot
  d PDA
  e Hypoplastic heart

3 A patient is admitted following a car crash, and is noted to have a haemothorax. Following insertion of a chest drain, what volume of blood loss would indicate referral for urgent surgical intervention?
  a 250 ml
  b 500 ml
  c 1000 ml
  d 1500 ml
  e 2000 ml

4 How many cusps does the mitral valve have?
  a 1
  b 2
  c 3
  d 4

5 Which of these vessels is not commonly used as a graft in CABG surgery?
  a Radial artery
  b Long saphenous vein
  c Brachial artery
  d Internal mammary artery
  e Short saphenous vein

6 What is the most likely location for an inhaled peanut to become lodged?
  a Right upper bronchus
  b Right middle bronchus
  c Right lower bronchus
  d Left upper bronchus
  e Left lower bronchus

7 What is the most common type of lung cancer?
  a Non-small cell carcinoma
  b Small cell carcinoma
  c Carcinoid
  d Sarcoma
  e Others

8 Which of the following is not a cause of cardiac tamponade?
  a Blunt trauma
  b Myocardial rupture
  c Pericarditis
  d Iatrogenic
  e Hyperthyroidism

9 An acute occlusion in the left anterior descending artery will cause the following ECG changes.
  a ST depression V1–V3
  b Left bundle branch block
  c ST elevation in V4–V6
  d ST elevation in II, III, aVF
  e ST elevation in V1–V3

10 Which of these is not an aspect of Tetralogy of Fallot?
 a   Pulmonary stenosis
 b   VSD
 c   PDA
 d   Overriding aorta
 e   Right ventricular hypertrophy

11 What suture material is used to close the sternum?
 a   Steel
 b   Prolene
 c   Silk
 d   Monocryl
 e   Vicryl

12 A patient is admitted following a car crash. He has fractured his left 9th rib. Which of the following organs is unlikely to be injured?
 a   Pancreas
 b   Spleen
 c   Liver
 d   Stomach
 e   Bladder

Answers

SAQs

1   a   True ribs 1–7
          False ribs 8–10
          Floating ribs 11–12
   b   Two adjacent ribs broken in at least two places.
   c   The flail segment moves in whilst the rest of the chest moves out (paradoxical movement).
   d   Ensure adequate oxygenation
          Analgesia – typically opiates are required
          Chest physiotherapy
          Regular deep breathing and coughing to prevent chest infections
   e   Pulmonary contusion

Any patient with a flail chest has had a significant force pass through their chest. They are much more likely to have a pneumothorax, haemothorax, or pulmonary contusion, and therefore require close observation.

2   a   Secure his airway
          Maintain cervical spine immobilisation
   b   Decreased chest wall movement
          Tracheal deviation
          Hyper-resonance to percussion
          Decreased vocal resonance/tactile fremitus
          Absence of breath sounds
   c   Insertion of a cannula to decompress the tension.
          Insert into the midclavicular line in the 2nd intercostal space.
   d   Chest drain insertion
          Insert in the triangle of safety, between the lateral border of pectoralis major, the anterior border of latissimus dorsi, above a line horizontal to the nipple, and below the axilla.

Tension pneumothorax is a life-threatening emergency which requires immediate treatment. It is caused by air under pressure in the pleural space, which occurs due to tissue forming a one way valve, allowing air in but not out.

3 a Observe – chest expansion, tracheal deviation, blunt or penetrating injuries, cyanosis

Palpate – pain indicating rib fracture, flail chest, tactile vocal fremitus

Percuss – dull, resonant, hyper-resonant

Auscultate – crepitations, decreased or absent breath sounds

  b 40%

  c A fluid level with a meniscus

  d Above the rib to avoid the neurovascular bundle.

  e Immediate drainage of more than 1500 ml.

Persistent drainage of more than 200 ml per hour for 2–4 hours.

A haemothorax is a collection of blood in the pleural space, which most commonly occurs due to trauma. The majority of cases resolve with conservative management, including insertion of a large bore chest drain and fluid replacement.

4 a Congestive heart failure

Syncope

Stroke

Ischaemic peripheral neuropathy

Paraplegia

Cardiac arrest

Sudden death

  b Hypertension

Connective tissue disorders

Marfan syndrome

Bicuspid aortic valve

Turner syndrome

Chest trauma

Cardiac surgery

Syphilis

Pregnancy

  c A widened mediastinum

  d 80%

  e Blood directly from an aortic rupture.

Fluid due to an inflammatory reaction around the aorta

Aortic dissection is usually a fatal condition, with 50% of patients not making it to hospital, and only 40% of those admitted surviving. It is a difficult diagnosis, mimicking MI. Patients should initially be managed medically by good blood pressure control, with surgical intervention required in acute dissections with organ failure, imminent rupture, or connective tissue disorders.

5 a Pectus excavatum
    b Pectus carinatum
    c Marfan's syndrome
    d There is a marked variation in the volume of breast tissue between males and females so it is often less prominent in females.
    e Body building to increase the pectoral muscle mass will often help to mask the condition.
    f Insertion of a specially designed steel bar underneath the sternum which is removed after 2–4 years.
    g Pain
       Bleeding
       Infection
       Scar
       Anaesthetic risks
       PE
       DVT
       Pneumothorax
       Recurrence
       Bar repositioning

Pectus excavatum and carinatum are both uncommon chest wall deformities. They tend not to cause any complications unless very pronounced, when they can inhibit breathing and cardiac function. Surgical intervention is painful and requires repeated procedures, therefore camouflage through awaiting breast development or increasing pectoral muscle mass is beneficial.

6 a Aortic stenosis
    b Dyspnoea
       Palpitations
       Chest pain
       Stroke
       Transient ischaemic attack
    c Bicuspid aortic valve
       Calcification of the aortic valve
       Rheumatic fever
    d Metallic valve – last approximately 20 years, but require lifelong warfarin
       Tissue valve – last approximately 10 years, but only requires warfarin for 6 months

Replacement heart valves may be either metallic or tissue depending upon the life expectancy of the patient, and other comorbidities. The surgery is typically done through a median sternotomy incision, however new techniques are developing to permit percutaneous valve replacement surgery.

7 a Transposition of the great arteries
Truncus arteriosus
Total anomalous pulmonary venous return
Hypoplastic left heart syndrome
Tricuspid atresia
  b Pulmonary stenosis
VSD
Overriding aorta
Right ventricular hypertrophy
  c Sudden death
Failure to thrive
Difficulty feeding
Poor weight gain
Developmental delay
Clubbing
  d Foramen ovale

Tetralogy of Fallot is present in 0.4 births per 1000. Untreated, 30% of patients survive 10 years. Surgery is carried out in patients less than 1 year-of-age with a less than 5% chance of mortality. The aim is to reduce the pulmonary stenosis and repair the VSD. These patients require life-long follow-up as they are at risk of heart failure, and pulmonary valve problems.

8 a Angina
  b Hypercholesterolaemia
Smoking
Male
Diabetes
Obesity
Family history under 50
Hypertension
Ethnicity
  c Diastole
  d Percutaneous intervention (stenting)
CABG
  e Coronary angiogram
  f Internal mammary artery
Radial artery
Long saphenous vein
Short saphenous vein

CABG surgery has become less common due to the role of percutaneous intervention, however, it remains a frequent treatment for multi-vessel and left anterior descending disease. The best results are from internal mammary or thoracic artery grafts.

9   a   From the pulmonary artery to the aortic arch

    b   Respiratory difficulty
       Poor growth
       Differential cyanosis
       Shortness of breath

    c   Continuous machinery like murmur
       Cardiomegaly
       Bounding pulse
       Widened pulse pressure
       Tachycardia
       Left subclavicular thrill

    d   Echocardiogram

    e   Medically – NSAIDs inhibit prostaglandin synthesis, permitting the duct to close
       Percutaneously – through coil embolisation or mesh occlusion
       Surgically – manually tying the duct

A PDA is more common in babies who are premature, have congenital rubella, or Down syndrome. The ductus arteriosus remains open allowing blood to pass from the aorta back around the lungs. Without treatment, the disease may progress to a right to left shunt (Eisenmenger syndrome) leading to cyanotic disease.

10   a   Horner's syndrome
       Hoarse voice
       Pain and weakness in the arm
       Superior vena cava syndrome

    b   Smoking
       Radon gas exposure
       Asbestos
       Viruses
       Family history
       Age

    c   Chemotherapy and radiotherapy

    d   Two

    e   Ten segments, three segments in the superior lobe, two in the middle lobe, and five in the inferior lobe.
       Each segment may be resected along with its blood and lymphatic supply to resect lung tumours.

Lung cancer accounts for over 1.3 million deaths worldwide per annum. It is typically differentiated into small cell and non-small cell, with non-small cell cancer more amenable to surgical resection. Patients may present with haemoptysis, chronic cough, weight loss, and signs related to compression of underlying structures.

11 a   Raised JVP
      Hypotension
      Muffled heart sounds
      Pulsus paradoxicus
      Tachycardia
    b   A large globular heart shadow
    c   FAST scan
    d   Pulseless ventricular tachycardia
      Ventricular fibrillation
    e   Pericardiocentesis – insert a large bore needle attached to a 20 ml syringe between the junction of the left costal margin and the xiphisternum, aiming at the left shoulder tip.

Cardiac tamponade typically occurs following blunt or penetrating trauma however it can occur due to hypothyroidism, pericarditis, or iatrogenically. Pericardiocentesis should be performed to relieve the tamponade, with a cannula left *in situ* in the trauma setting. Surgical intervention may be required to form a pericardial window, and stop the source of bleeding.

EMQs

1	**G**	10	**B**	19	**H**	
2	**A**	11	**D**	20	**C**	
3	**B**	12	**C**	21	**C**	
4	**D**	13	**B**	22	**A**	
5	**C**	14	**E**	23	**D**	
6	**E**	15	**A**	24	**G**	
7	**A**	16	**A**	25	**E**	
8	**C**	17	**E**			
9	**D**	18	**G**			

MCQs

1   e – A tension pneumothorax is an emergency, requiring immediate decompression on clinical grounds, prior to a chest X-ray. You may notice tracheal deviation, rapid shallow breaths, low sats, decreased chest expansion, hyper-resonance to percussion, and an absence of breath sounds. A cannula should be inserted into the midclavicular line 2nd intercostal space immediately, with a chest drain inserted following this.

2   b – AVSDs are the most common cardiac abnormality in Down syndrome (45%), with VSDs in 35%, atrial septal defects in 8%, PDA 7%, and Fallot's tetralogy 4-6%.

3   d – Any haemothorax which drains more than 1500 ml immediately following chest drain insertion, or persistent drainage of more than 200 ml per hour for 2–4 hours requires urgent surgical intervention. A smaller haemothorax can be managed with regular blood tests and observation, with a chest drain inserted until bleeding stops.

4   b – The mitral valve is bicuspid, and lies between the left atrium and ventricle. The tricuspid valve has three cusps.

5   c – The others are all used commonly for grafts in a CABG. Prior to using the radial artery one should perform Allen's test, by occluding the radial and ulnar arteries and pumping the hand to drain the blood for 30 seconds. The ulnar artery should then be released to ensure the hand become pink within 7 seconds. This ensures that the blood supply to the hand is sufficient from the ulnar artery alone.

6   b – An inhaled peanut is most likely to become lodged in the right middle bronchus as the right main bronchus is wider, shorter and more vertical than the left main bronchus, and the right middle bronchus is wider than the lower bronchus.

7   a – Non small cell lung cancer accounts for just under 80% of lung cancers, and are potentially resectable. Small cell lung carcinoma accounts for just under 20% of lung cancers, and is typically treated with chemoradiotherapy. Carcinoid accounts for 1%, sarcoid 0.1%, and others 2%.

8   e – Hypothyroidism not hyperthyroidism may cause cardiac tamponade.

9   d – The left anterior descending artery supplies blood to the ventricular septum, apex, and anterolateral myocardium. Occlusion typically causes an anterior MI, with ST elevation in leads II, III, and aVF.

10   c – A PDA is not associated with Fallot's tetralogy.

11   a – The sternum is very tough, and takes a long time to heal, therefore a very strong non absorbable material (steel) is used for this closure. This leaves characteristic signs on chest X-ray.

12   e – Rib fractures can injure not only the lungs, but also the intra-abdominal organs.

Chapter 12

Maxillofacial surgery

Philip Stather

SAQs

1   An 18-year-old man was admitted following a brawl. He reports that he was kicked in the head, and now has difficulty opening his mouth. He has also vomited twice, and says that he blacked out during the assault.
   a   How will you protect his cervical spine until it is cleared?   (3 marks)
   b   List the five aspects of a neurological examination.   (5 marks)
   c   Give three indications for CT head following head trauma.   (3 marks)
   d   On examination, he has tenderness over the right mandible. What further imaging would you like to arrange?   (1 mark)
   e   This reveals a non-displaced fracture of the right mandible. What else should you look for in relation to this?   (1 mark)

2   A 35-year-old lady comes to your GP surgery complaining of pain when chewing, radiating around her jaw, and is unable to open her mouth wide, with a grating sound upon movement of the jaw.
   a   What bone does the mandible articulate with?   (1 mark)
   b   Which nerve passes through the mandibular foramen?   (1 mark)
   c   Name the three muscles of mastication.   (3 marks)
   d   Give two further symptoms this patient may suffer from.   (2 marks)
   e   What is the name of this condition?   (1 mark)
   f   Give two possible causes of this condition.   (2 marks)
   g   Give two treatment options for this condition.   (2 marks)

3   A 40-year-old overweight gentleman comes to see you as he says he is tired all the time. He feels that despite going to bed early he is tossing and turning all night, and in he morning, feels like he has not slept. His partner reports that he snores.

a   What is the most likely diagnosis?   (1 mark)
b   Name the scoring system used for this condition, and
     list two of the questions in this system.   (3 marks)
c   Apart from snoring and sleepiness give two further
     symptoms of this condition.   (2 marks)
d   Name one investigation you can request for diagnosis.   (1 mark)
e   Give three lifestyle changes which can help with this
     condition.   (3 marks)
f   Give two further treatment options.   (2 marks)

4   A 30-year-old man is brought in to A&E following a road traffic collision
      (RTC), where his face hit the dashboard. On admission, his GCS is 7.
      On examination, he has mobility of his upper teeth, malocclusion, and
      swelling of the upper lip.
a   What protocol will you use to assess and treat this
     patient, and describe the first three aspects of your
     immediate management.   (4 marks)
b   Following initial stabilisation you arrange a CT scan
     which shows no spinal fractures, and no intracranial
     pathology, however he is noted to have a facial fracture.
     What is the classification system used for facial fractures? (1 mark)
c   His fracture involves the maxillary sinus. Name the
     three other sinuses in the skull.   (3 marks)
d   What treatment is required regarding his facial fracture?   (2 marks)

5   A 63-year-old lady comes to see you regarding pain in her tooth. You
      suspect she has a dental abscess.
a   Give three further symptoms you would ask about.   (3 marks)
b   What is the treatment of an abscess?   (1 mark)
c   In a patient who has recurrent abscesses list three
     further conditions you should enquire about.   (3 marks)
d   If the abscess is not treated give three complications
     which may potentially occur.   (3 marks)

6   A 26-year-old lady comes to see you regarding pain over her left cheek,
      following coryzal symptoms the previous week.
a   What is the most likely diagnosis?   (1 mark)
b   Name two of the most common causative agents.   (2 marks)
c   When will you give patients antibiotics for this condition? (1 mark)
d   List three risk factors for this condition.   (3 marks)
e   Give two forms of conservative treatment for the
     chronic form of this condition.   (2 marks)
f   Name the surgical intervention for the chronic form of
     this condition.   (1 mark)

7 You are referred a young baby who has a congenital cleft palate.

   a Explain the difference between complete and
incomplete cleft palate. (2 marks)

   b What is the incidence of this condition? (1 mark)

   c Without surgical intervention suggest three difficulties
the baby may encounter. (3 marks)

   d At what age is this condition usually corrected? (1 mark)

   e How may the uvula differ in this patient? (1 mark)

   f Give two risk factors for developing cleft lip. (2 marks)

8 A 25-year-old lady is admitted with a swelling in the parotid gland. On
examination, she has a stone blocking the duct.

   a Explain the differences in saliva between the different
salivary glands. (3 marks)

   b Which nerve passes through the parotid gland? (1 mark)

   c Where does the parotid drain do, and what is the name
of this duct? (2 marks)

   d Give three functions of saliva. (3 marks)

   e Give two treatments for salivary duct stones. (2 marks)

9 A 50-year-old man presents with a white patch on the side of his tongue
which is hairy in appearance.

   a Explain the innervation of the tongue. (3 marks)

   b Name three extrinsic muscles of the tongue. (3 marks)

   c You suspect oral hairy leukoplakia. Give two groups of
patients who are at a higher risk of this condition. (2 marks)

   d What is the virus implicated in this condition? (1 mark)

   e Suggest a treatment option for this patient. (1 mark)

10 A 10-year-old boy is seen in clinic due to multiple problems with his
teeth. He has extensive tooth decay.

   a What is the medical term for this condition? (1 mark)

   b What is the outer layer of the tooth? (1 mark)

   c Which teeth does this commonly affect in this age group? (1 mark)

   d Give three life style modifications you should suggest to
the patient. (3 marks)

   e How many baby teeth does the average person have? (1 mark)

   f At what age do the lower two incisors erupt? (1 mark)

   g This patient undergoes extraction of multiple teeth due
to his decay. Give three complications of this procedure. (3 marks)

EMQs

Match the description to the diagnosis:

A Oral hairy leukoplakia
B Squamous cell carcinoma (SCC)
C Geographic tongue
D Oral candidiasis
E Lichen planus

1 An opportunistic fungal infection more common in immunosuppressed patients.
2 A white patch on the side of the tongue with a corrugated appearance.
3 An inflammatory condition with tongue cracking.
4 Pruritic, planar, purple, polygonal papules.
5 A rapidly spreading malignant lesion.

At what age do the following teeth commonly erupt?

A 6 months
B 1 year
C 18 months
D 2 years
E 3 years
F 6 years
G 8 years
H 13 years

6 1st tooth
7 1st canine
8 Second molar
9 Permanent central incisor
10 Permanent second molar

What imaging would you recommend in each case?
A Nil
B X-ray
C USS
D CT
E MRI
F PET
G Sialography

11 A patient with chronic recurrent sinusitis.
12 A patient admitted following RTC with a GCS 11.
13 A patient admitted following a brawl with difficulty opening his mouth.
14 A patient with swelling of the parotid gland and a hard lump inside the cheek.
15 A pregnant lady with a large spreading SCC on her tongue.

Which nerve fits the description below?
A Trigeminal nerve
B Facial nerve
C Mental nerve
D Inferior alveolar nerve
E Auriculotemporal nerve
F Glossopharyngeal nerve
G Vagus nerve

16 Travels through the mandibular canal.
17 Supplies the muscles of mastication.
18 Supplies the posterior third of the tongue.
19 Divides into its branches in the parotid gland.
20 Give off the recurrent laryngeal nerve.

Calculate the GCS for each patient.
A 0
B 3
C 6
D 7
E 9
F 13
G 15

21 Eyes not opening, incomprehensible sounds, abnormal flexion to pain.
22 An alert patient who is talking with coherent but slurred speech, the eye is drooping on the left, and she has weakness in her left arm.

23 Moribund patient.

24 Eyes opening to voice, confused speech, obeying commands.

25 Eyes open to pain, uttering inappropriate words in response to pain, withdrawal to painful stimuli.

MCQs

1 Which statement is true regarding the parotid gland?
- a   It is a mucous salivary gland
- b   It is found wrapped around the mandibular ramus
- c   The internal carotid artery passes through the gland
- d   Empties opposite the 2nd lower molar tooth
- e   Has parasympathetic innervation from the facial nerve

2 A gentleman is admitted following an RTC. He is opening his eyes to pain, and uttering inappropriate words. He also localises to your painful stimulus. Calculate his GCS.
- a   15
- b   12
- c   10
- d   8
- e   5

3 On average, at what age do permanent teeth begin to erupt?
- a   4
- b   5
- c   6
- d   7
- e   8

4 Which nerve supplies sensation to the lower lip?
- a   Mental nerve
- b   Trigeminal nerve
- c   Inferior alveolar nerve
- d   Facial nerve
- e   Glossopharyngeal nerve

5 Which of the following is not a cause of gingival hypertrophy?
- a   Anticonvulsant therapy
- b   Cyclosporine
- c   Pregnancy
- d   Leukaemia
- e   Hyperthyroidism

6 Which of the following is not a symptom of malocclusion?
  a Abnormal alignment of teeth
  b Speech difficulties
  c Mouth breathing
  d Headache
  e Difficulty in mastication

7 Into which structure does the maxillary sinus drain?
  a The superior meatus
  b The middle meatus
  c The inferior meatus
  d The sphenoethmoidal recess

8 Which of the following is not a risk factor for obstructive sleep apnoea (OSA)?
  a Obesity
  b Neck circumference > 17 inches
  c Male
  d Alcohol
  e Day time somnolence

9 What excision margin should be used for a malignant melanoma <1 mm depth?
  a 1 mm
  b 5 mm
  c 10 mm
  d 15 mm
  e 20 mm

10 Which statement is true regarding nasal fracture?
  a All patients with nasal fracture require manipulation
  b Manipulation can be done up to 2 months following injury
  c Manipulation restores the nose to its previous shape
  d Patients may present with an obstructed nostril
  e Septal haematoma can be treated conservatively

Answers

SAQs

1 a Blocks
        Collar
        Tape
     b Tone
        Power
        Reflexes
        Sensation
        Co-ordination
     c GCS <13 at any point since injury
        GCS = 13 or 14 at 2 hours after injury
        Suspected open basal skull fracture.
        More than one episode of vomiting in patients >12 years of age.
        Aged over 65 years with some loss of consciousness or amnesia.
        Focal neurological defect.
        Amnesia for more than 30 minutes.
        Dangerous mechanism of injury.
     d X-rays (facial views)
     e A second fracture as the mandible frequently fractures in two places
        at once.

Head trauma is a very common presentation to A&E, and it is often difficult to determine whether patients have had significant head trauma or are intoxicated. Until their cervical spine is cleared they should have three-point immobilisation.

Mandibular fractures often occur in two locations, therefore it is important to look for a second fracture in these patients.

2 a Temporal bone
     b Inferior alveolar nerve
     c Masseter
        Temporalis
        Medial and lateral pterygoids
     d Earache
        Headache
        Tinnitus
     e Temperomandibular joint (TMJ) dysfunction

    f   Trauma
        Clenching or grinding of teeth
        Jaw thrusting
        Arthritis
        Malalignment of teeth
    g   Analgesia
        Joint irrigation
        Mouth guards
        Surgical repositioning of the jaw

TMJ dysfunction typically presents with pain, restricted jaw movement, and joint noise. It is useful to measure the distance between incisors, and ensure the pain is not coming from the salivary glands, oral cavity, cranial nerves or ears.

3   **a**   OSA
    b   Epworth sleepiness scale. Using the following scale please choose the most appropriate number for each situation. 0 = would never doze or sleep, 1 = slight chance of dozing or sleeping, 2 = moderate chance of dozing or sleeping, 3 = high chance of dozing or sleeping:
- sitting and reading
- watching TV
- sitting inactive in a public space
- being a passenger in a motor vehicle for an hour
- lying down in the afternoon
- sitting and talking to someone
- sitting quietly after lunch (no alcohol)
- stopping for a few minutes in traffic while driving.

    c   Morning headaches
        Insomnia
        Mood changes
        Poor concentration
        Irritability
        Anxiety
        Depression
        Hypertension
        Obesity
    d   Sleep studies
        Polysomnography
        Home oximetry
    e   Weight loss
        Stopping smoking
        Avoiding alcohol

f   Continuous positive airway pressure (CPAP)
Surgical intervention (tonsillectomy, adenoidectomy, maxillomandibular advancement)

OSA is a sleeping pattern whereby people have abnormal pauses in their breathing, leading to hypoxia and wakening. They typically have daytime somnolence, and loud snoring. It is more common in people who are overweight, elderly, smokers, or diabetics.

4 **a** ATLS
Cervical spine immobilisation
Oxygen
Airway protection through intubation as GCS < 8
    b Le Fort
    c Frontal
Sphenoid
Ethmoid
    d Surgical intervention
Antibiotics as it is considered an open fracture

There are three types of Le Fort fracture. A Le Fort I fracture is a horizontal fracture through the maxilla. A Le Fort II fracture is pyramidal through the nasal bridge and frontal processes of the maxilla. A Le Fort III fracture is through the nasal bridge, orbits, sphenoid, ethmoid, and zygomatic arches.

5 **a** Swelling or tenderness of the gum
Swelling of the face
Loose tooth
Fever
Difficulty eating or swallowing
    b Incision and drainage
    c Diabetes
HIV
Chemotherapy
Splenectomy
Any medical condition requiring long term steroid treatment
    d Abscess may burst creating a sinus tract
OM
Sinusitis
Dental cyst
Cavernous sinus thrombosis
Ludwig's angina

Dental abscesses typically present with pain, gum tenderness and swelling, facial swelling, fever, and a loose tooth. Treatment is through draining the pus either by lancing the abscess or drilling a hole in the tooth. It is important to reinforce a healthy diet and brushing of the teeth.

6   a   Acute sinusitis
     b   *Streptococcus pneumonia*
         Haemophilus influenza
         Moraxella catarrhalis
         Viral
     c   Most cases are viral therefore will resolve within 7 days
         Antibiotics can be used for persistent infections or very severe systemic symptoms.
     d   URTI
         Dental infection
         Allergic rhinitis
         Anatomical variations
         Asthma
         Cystic fibrosis
         Smoking
         Pregnancy
         Inflammatory conditions
         Immunodeficiency
     e   Nasal irrigation
         Nasal decongestant sprays
         Intranasal corticosteroids
     f   FESS

Acute sinusitis typically occurs after an URTI, leading to a viral infection in the sinus. It usually resolves within 1 week, however it may continue for up to 12 weeks. The aim of treatment is to encourage the infection to drain out of the sinuses by nasal decongestants and irrigation, with antibiotics reserved for those patients not responding to these treatments.

7   a   Complete includes the soft and hard palate.
         Incomplete is a hole in the roof of the mouth usually a cleft soft palate.
     b   1 in 700
     c   Difficulty feeding
         Ear disease
         Speech difficulties
         Hearing difficulties
         Psychosocial issues

  d Typically at 10 weeks old, when the baby weighs 4.5 kg, and has a haemoglobin of 10.

  e Bifid uvula

  f Genetics

     Environmental – maternal smoking, alcohol, obesity, lack of folic acid, medications

Cleft lip and palate occurs in 1 in 700 babies, and is due to a failure of fusion of the maxillary and medial nasal processes. It can cause problems with feeding, speech, and hearing, and requires surgical correction at 10 weeks of age.

8 **a** Parotid gland – serous

     Submandibular gland – mixed serous and mucous

     Sublingual gland – mucous

  b Facial nerve

  c Opposite the second upper molar tooth

     Stenson's duct/parotid duct

  d Moistening food

     Creation of bolus

     Digestion of carbohydrates

     Disinfectant

     Hormonal – secretion of Gustin hormone which plays a role in the development of taste buds

  e Gentle probing into the duct

     Therapeutic sialendoscopy

     Shockwave treatment

     Surgical removal

Patients with stones in the parotid ducts often present with intermittent pain and swelling in the gland, with a palpable stone in the duct. This condition often settles on passing of the stones, which may be aided by gentle manipulation in clinic.

9 **a** Anterior 2/3 – chorda tympani (facial nerve) for taste, lingual nerve (trigeminal) for sensation

     Posterior 1/3 – Glossopharyngeal nerve

  b Genioglossus

     Hyoglossus

     Styloglossus

     Palatoglossus

  c HIV

     Immunosuppressed patients

     Patients on steroids

    d   EBV
    e   Observation only
         Antiviral therapy (acyclovir) may be used

Oral hairy leukoplakia is a white patch on the side of the tongue more commonly seen in immunocompromised patients. It usually resolves spontaneously.

10 a   Dental caries
      b   Enamel
      c   Incisors
      d   Fewer sweets
         Avoid cola and sugary drinks
         Regular tooth brushing
         Regular visits to the dentist
         Floss
      e   20
      f   6 months
      g   Pain
         Bleeding
         Oozing
         Infection
         Dry socket
         Swelling
         Nerve injury

Tooth decay is a process whereby bacteria erode the hard tooth structures such as enamel, dentin, and cementum. It is exacerbated by sugary drinks and sweets, with good oral hygiene and dietary modification the mainstay of treatment.

EMQs

1	**D**	10	**H**	19	**B**
2	**A**	11	**D**	20	**G**
3	**C**	12	**D**	21	**C**
4	**E**	13	**B**	22	**G**
5	**B**	14	**G**	23	**B**
6	**A**	15	**E**	24	**F**
7	**C**	16	**D**	25	**E**
8	**D**	17	**A**		
9	**G**	18	**F**		

MCQs

1 b – The parotid gland is located overlying the mandibular ramus, anterior and inferior to the external ear. The facial nerve and its branches, the external carotid artery, and the retromandibular vein pass through the gland. It empties opposite the 2nd upper molar tooth.

2 d – Eyes 2, Verbal 3, Motor 5.

3 c – Permanent teeth begin to erupt around 6 years-of-age, initially with the first molars. The process is usually complete by 13 years-of-age, apart from the wisdom teeth.

4 a – The mandibular branch of the trigeminal nerve gives off the inferior alveolar branch, which enters the mandibular foramen and travels through the mandibular canal. At the mental foramen it divides into the incisive nerve and mental nerve. The incisive nerve supplies the anterior teeth, whilst the mental nerve supplies the lower lip.

5 e – Gingival hypertrophy typically occurs due to chronic inflammation, anticonvulsants, calcium channel blockers, cyclosporine, pregnancy, puberty, vitamin C deficiency, leukaemia, granulomatous disease, and neoplastic lesions.

6 d – Malocclusion can be differentiated into prognathism (underbite) or retrognathism (overbite). It is commonly treated with braces, however in severe forms mandibular advancement may be required.

7 b – The superior meatus communicates with the posterior ethmoid air cells, the middle meatus communicates with the frontal sinus, maxillary sinus, and anterior ethmoid air cells, the inferior meatus communicates with the nasolacrimal canal, and the sphenoethmoidal recess communicates with the sphenoid sinus.

8 e – Day time somnolence is a symptom of OSA. The risk factors include being male, overweight, large neck circumference, hypertension, narrowed airway, age, family history, alcohol, smoking, and prolonged sitting.

9 c – 5 mm margins are recommended for melanoma *in situ*, 1 cm for <1 mm depth, and 20 mm for deeper tumours.

10 d – Nasal fractures typically present with pain and deformity, associated with swelling and possible nasal occlusion due to septal deviation or haematoma. In cases where there is minimal displacement this may be treated conservatively. When manipulation is required this should be done within 2 weeks of the injury.

Chapter 13

Neurosurgery

Alexander Rawlinson

SAQs

1 A 10-ten-month old girl is referred to the neurosurgical out-patient clinic by a GP with a history of increasing head circumference, outside of normal parameters, and failure to thrive.

   a What is the most likely diagnosis? (1 mark)

   b What is the most common congenital anatomical cause of this condition? (1 mark)

   c Give one classification for this condition. (1 mark)

   d What congenital central nervous system (CNS) disorder is often associated with this clinical presentation? (1 mark)

   e Give the clinical findings you may expect on examination. (3 marks)

   f What investigation may be performed in order to confirm the diagnosis? (1 mark)

   g What is the possible management option in this patient, and explain how it works? (2 marks)

2 A 27-year-old motorcyclist is brought to A&E following a collision with a car. He complains of not being able to move his legs. His GCS is 15 throughout and there are no obvious signs of significant blood loss. He has a pulse rate of 45 bpm and blood pressure of 85/40 mmHg.

   a What is your initial diagnosis? (1 mark)

   b Give two common causes of this condition. (2 marks)

   c What is the underlying neurological deficit? (1 mark)

   d How can the haemodynamic status of this patient be explained? (3 marks)

   e What role do fluids and vasopressors have in the management of this patient? (2 marks)

   f How does this condition contrast to spinal shock? (1 mark)

3 A 72-year-old fell down a flight of stairs. Clinical examination reveals weakness in the upper limbs and normal power in the legs. She has paraesthesia throughout the upper limbs.

   a What is your initial diagnosis? (1 mark)

   b What is the usual mechanism of injury? (1 mark)

c Give two structures which may compress the cord. (2 marks)
d Give two other conditions which are associated with this
   presentation. (2 marks)
e Compare this condition with anterior cord syndrome. (3 marks)
f What vascular structure is compromised in anterior
   cord syndrome? (1 mark)

4 A 57-year-old businessman collapses on the golf course. On arrival in
   A&E his playing partner describes witnessing a tonic-clonic seizure. On
   review, the patient's GCS is 15. He admits to a 3-month history of severe
   headaches and lethargy, which he attributed to stress. Neurological
   examination is unremarkable apart from bilateral papilloedema.
   a What is at the top of your list of differential diagnoses? (1 mark)
   b Explain the Monro-Kelly Doctrine. (3 marks)
   c What intracranial processes cause papilloedema? (3 marks)
   d As a teaching point, the A&E consultant asks whether
      you should perform a lumbar puncture on this patient.
      What is your response? (2 marks)
   e After routine bloods and X-ray, what would be your
      investigation of choice to aid diagnosis? (1 mark)

5 A 42-year-old woman presents with a severe, post-coital occipital
   headache. She describes the initial sensation like 'being hit on the back of
   the head with a baseball bat'.
   a What is your initial diagnosis? (1 mark)
   b Give three pathophysiological processes which may
      cause this. (3 marks)
   c In addition to severe headache, give two other
      symptoms the patient may present with and which other
      condition should be excluded? (2 marks)
   d Give two investigations you would perform in order to
      confirm this diagnosis (2 marks)
   e Name two intracerebral vessels commonly implicated in
      the diagnosis. (2 marks)

6 A 26-year-old male is brought to A&E with a GCS of 7 after being
   involved in a fight outside the local pub. His girlfriend describes a brief
   loss of consciousness which then resolved. On their return home, he
   became progressively drowsy and confused.
   a What would be your most likely differential diagnosis? (1 mark)
   b What area of the skull is commonly fractured in
      association with this presentation, and which blood
      vessel is injured? (2 marks)
   c A CT brain is performed. What is the classical
      radiological appearance? (2 marks)

   d Give three findings which may be present on
neurological examination and how may they be
explained? (3 marks)

   e Outline the initial management of this patient. (2 marks)

7 A 63-year-old with a past history of excess alcohol intake presents with
worsening headache and drowsiness. She is a vague historian but her
husband informs you that she has had several falls recently. CT scan
reveals a large, crescent-shaped hypodense area between the inner table
of the skull and the surface of the left cerebral hemisphere.

   a What is the most likely diagnosis? (1 mark)

   b How do you know whether this is a chronic or acute
event? (2 marks)

   c What is the pathophysiological cause of this
presentation? (2 marks)

   d Give four signs or symptoms you may find on
examination. (4 marks)

   e What surgical intervention may this patient require? (1 mark)

8 A 37-year-old IV drug user presents with headache, rigors and intermittent
tonic-clonic seizures. She describes a 6-month history of chronic upper
respiratory tract symptoms and purulent nasal discharge.

   a What is your initial diagnosis? (1 mark)

   b Following routine baseline investigations, what would
be your investigation of choice to confirm this diagnosis? (1 mark)

   c Would you perform a lumbar puncture in this patient?
Give reasons for your answer. (2 marks)

   d Give three further clinical findings you may discover
that support your diagnosis. (3 marks)

   e What are the possible causative organisms involved and
outline a broad management plan? (3 marks)

9 A 42-year-old woman is referred to clinic with headache and visual
disturbance. She states that she has recently had to buy new shoes
and gloves due to increasing hands and feet size. Blood tests reveal a
significantly elevated growth hormone level.

   a What is your initial diagnosis? What imaging would you
perform to confirm the diagnosis? (2 marks)

   b What is the name of this presenting syndrome? (1 mark)

   c What visual field deficit would you expect to find on
examination and what is the cause? (2 marks)

   d In addition to the visual field deficit, what else may you
find on examination of the eyes? (2 marks)

   e In addition to growth hormone, which other hormones
are produced by this gland? (3 marks)

10 A 19-year-old female presents to A&E having suffered a penetrating knife injury to the back. She is unable to move her right leg and is complaining of severe pain in the right leg having suffered a second knife injury. She has no temperature sensation in the left leg.

    a   What is your initial diagnosis?   (1 mark)

    b   What is the explanation for these findings?   (4 marks)

    c   Which tracts are responsible for motor and proprioception/touch fibres?   (2 marks)

    d   In addition to trauma, give two possible other causes of this clinical presentation.   (2 marks)

    e   What would be the imaging modality of choice to confirm this diagnosis?   (1 mark)

EMQs

For each of the scenarios below select the appropriate diagnosis from the following list:

A Subdural haematoma
B Open skull fracture
C Axonal brain injury
D Scalp haematoma
E Subarachnoid haemorrhage (SAH)
F Compound skull fracture
G Subaponeurotic haematoma
H Extradural haematoma
I Base of skull fracture
J Concussion

1 A 72-year-old with dementia is brought to A&E with right-sided hemiparesis. His wife tells you he slipped and banged his head 8 days ago. He has been complaining of headaches and has become more confused. He is warfarinised due to atrial fibrillation.

2 A 19-year-old presents to A&E after being hit on the side of the head with a golf club. His friend states that he was knocked out for approximately 30 seconds but on presentation his GCS is 15. A plain X-ray of the skull reveals a fracture in the region of the left parietal area. Whilst still in A&E his GCS suddenly falls to 6.

3 A 32-year-old cyclist is brought to A&E by the paramedics after being knocked off his bike by a lorry. His GCS is 8 and you note clear fluid coming out of his nose and right ear.

4 A 17-year-old fan of wrestling presents with a bilateral diffuse, fluctuant swelling of the scalp after being dropped on his head during his lunch hour 3 days ago. He reports no loss of consciousness or fluid loss from either the nose or ears.

5 A 52-year-old woman presents with sudden onset occipital headache. She describes an initial sensation of being hit around the back of the head. On examination, she has neck stiffness and photophobia.

For the scenarios detailed below, select the most appropriate diagnosis from the following list:

A Subdural haematoma
B Intraventricular haemorrhage
C Base of skull fracture
D Le Fort I fracture
E Le Fort II fracture
F Extradural haematoma
G Diffuse axonal injury
H Intracerebral haemorrhage

6 A 23-year-old cyclist collides with a lamppost sustaining facial injuries. There is significant facial swelling and an associated haematoma. A subsequent CT scan shows a low-level horizontal fracture of the maxilla extending above the maxillary teeth. It passes low down in the maxilla around the level of the nasal floor and maxillary sinus and extends back through the pterygoid plates. There is no evidence of skull base involvement.

7 A 42-year-old window cleaner has fallen from the top of his ladder. On arrival in A&E he has a GCS of 3. A CT brain is reported as showing minimal differentiation between the grey and white matter, effacement of both lateral ventricles and loss of the normal sulcal pattern.

8 A 28-year-old nightclub doorman presents to A&E after being assaulted. On examination, there is bilateral periorbital haematomas and bruising over the right mastoid process. His GCS has remained 15 since the incident.

9 A 16-year-old opening batsman was hit on the side of the head by the cricket ball, whilst wearing no helmet. This caused him to lose consciousness for about 60 seconds but his GCS subsequently recovered to 15. Whilst waiting for a skull X-ray in A&E he becomes drowsy and confused.

10 A 25-year-old cyclist collides with a lamppost sustaining facial injuries. A CT reconstruction scan reveals a pyramidal fracture that extends from the pterygoid plates across the infraorbital rims and up to the nasofrontal junction.

For the following neurological observations, select the appropriate GCS score from the list below:

A GCS 4
B GCS 5
C GCS 6
D GCS 7
E GCS 8
F GCS 9
G GCS 10
H GCS 11
I GCS 12
J GCS 13

11 Eye opening to speech, localises to pain, confused speech.
12 Eye opening to pain, normal flexion to pain, incomprehensible sounds.
13 Eye opening spontaneously, obeys command, inappropriate words.
14 Eye opening spontaneously, abnormal flexion to pain, incomprehensible sounds.
15 Eye opening spontaneously, normal flexion to pain, inappropriate words.

For each of the following clinical scenarios, choose the most appropriate management option from the list below:

A CT head
B Intubation and ventilation
C Skull X-ray
D Admission for neurological observation
E Home with advice
F Referral to neurosurgical service
G Emergency burr-hole evacuation in A&E
H MRI head
I Lumbar puncture
J IV Mannitol

16 A 76-year-old woman who is on warfarin presents with a scalp laceration following a fall. Her GCS remains 15 throughout and she lives with her daughter.
17 A 22-year-old male is assaulted with a crowbar. Investigations reveal a depressed skull fracture.
18 A 52-year-old woman has a brief loss of consciousness after banging her head on a car door. She cannot recall the event but remembers everything since regaining consciousness. She lives at home with her adult daughter.

19 A 19-year-old male is involved in an RTA. His GCS remains 15
P throughout but he is noted to have clear fluid coming from his nose.

20 A 27-year-old woman presents complaining of severe headache. Whilst taking the history her GCS deteriorates to 7.

For the following clinical scenarios, choose the appropriate diagnosis from the list below:

A Posterior cord syndrome
B Cervical spondylosis
C Prolapsed L4 intervertebral disc
D Prolapsed L5 intervertebral disc
E Cauda equina syndrome
F Central cord syndrome
G Anterior cord syndrome
H Spinal cord transaction
I Brown-Sequard syndrome
J Cerebrovascular accident

21 An 80-year-old woman with known cervical spondylosis presents with flaccid weakness in both arms following a fall. On neurological examination, both legs are normal.

22 A 59-year-old woman falls onto her coccyx whilst walking down the
G stairs. On neurological examination, she has no power in the left leg with loss of pain and temperature sensation. Sensation to touch is preserved.

23 A 23-year-old man falls head first from his ladder, hyperextending his
A neck. On neurological examination, there is loss of proprioception, but power and sensation remain intact.

24 A 27-year-old man receives a stab wound to the back during a fight.
I On neurological examination, there is loss of power, fine touch and proprioception in the left leg. There is loss of temperature sensation in the right leg.

25 A 47-year-old presents with a 4-hour history of bilateral leg pain. She has
E had one episode of urinary incontinence. On examination, there is saddle paraesthesia and loss of anal tone.

MCQs

1 The GCS incorporates assessment of which of the following:
a Power assessment of the upper limbs
b Babinski response
c Pupil reactivity to light
d Verbal response
e Heart rate

2 A 52-year-old lorry driver presents with a severe, sudden onset headache which required him to pull over onto the hard shoulder. There is no relief with analgesia and no history of trauma. In A&E, his GCS deteriorates requiring intubation and ventilation. CT scan reveals dilatation of the lateral ventricles and intraventricular blood. What is the most likely diagnosis?
a Chronic subdural haemorrhage
b Acute subdural haemorrhage
c Extradural haemorrhage
d SAH
e Diffuse axonal injury

3 A 17-year-old competitive BMX rider is brought to A&E following a fall from his bike. The event doctor describes witnessing hyperextension of the neck. On examination, the rider has an ataxic gait. What is the likely diagnosis?
a Brown-Sequard syndrome
b Anterior cord syndrome
c Central cord syndrome
d Cauda equina syndrome
e Posterior cord syndrome

4 Which of the following clinical presentations should alert you to the possibility of base of skull fracture:
a T wave inversion on ECG
b Hemiplegia
c Radiculopathy in the upper limbs
d Subconjunctival haemorrhage
e Anosmia

5 A 19-year-old is brought to A&E after being involved in a fight. He smells strongly of cannabis. On examination, his GCS is 14 (confused speech). A CT scan reveals areas of haemorrhage in the fronto-temporal regions bilaterally. Twelve hours later, the nursing staff call you to say that his GCS has deteriorated to 11 (E2 V3 M6). What is the most likely diagnosis?
a   Chronic subdural haematoma
b   Extradural haemorrhage
c   Cerebral contusion
d   Acute subdural haematoma
e   Base of skull fracture

6 A 46-year-old woman presents to her GP with a left sided ptosis and dilated pupil. Which cranial nerve is involved?
a   Facial nerve
b   Oculomotor nerve
c   Optic nerve
d   Trigeminal nerve
e   Abducent nerve

7 A 79-year-old man is brought to A&E by his wife due to increased confusion. There is a history of a fall 48 hours ago. CT brain reveals a hyperdense concave area against the inner aspect of the right fronto-temporal region of the skull. What is the likely diagnosis?
a   Chronic subdural haematoma
b   Extradural haemorrhage
c   SOL
d   Acute subdural haematoma
e   Cerebral contusions

8 Regarding cerebral tumours, which of the following statements is correct?
a   The peak incidence of astrocytoma is in the elderly
b   Medulloblastoma is the commonest glioma in middle age
c   Meningiomas arise from arachnoid cells
d   Glioblastoma multiforme is a benign condition
e   In acoustic neuroma, tinnitus is an uncommon presenting symptom

9 A 37-year-old woman presents to A&E with headache, rigors, swelling and paralysis of movement in the right eye. She has recently completed a course of antibiotics prescribed for sinusitis. What is the likely diagnosis?
   a   Intra-cranial SOL
   b   Cavernous sinus thrombosis
   c   Uveitis
   d   Chronic sinusitis
   e   Sigmoid sinus thrombosis

10 A 22-year-old male is brought to A&E following a fall from a third floor window. He has a GCS of 3. On examination, you note that all four limbs are flaccid and you are unable to elicit any reflexes. You note that the patient has a paradoxical breathing pattern. What is the likely site of injury?
   a   Cervical cord
   b   Spinothalamic tract
   c   Cauda equina
   d   Corticospinal tract
   e   Middle meningeal artery

Answers

SAQs

1 a Hydrocephalus
   b Aqueduct of Sylvius stenosis/cerebral aqueduct stensosis.
   c Communicating or non-communicating
      Congenital or acquired
   d Spina bifida
   e Head circumference that is beyond normal parameters when
      compared with growth charts.
      Dilated scalp veins.
      A tense anterior fontanelle.
      Setting sun appearance of the eyes.
      A lethargic, irritable infant.
   f MR brain (CT is an alternative but high radiation dose)
   g A ventriculo-peritoneal shunt may be inserted between the lateral
      ventricle and peritoneal cavity. It consists of a one-way valve which
      allows cerebrospinal fluid (CSF) to drain from the ventricular
      system into the peritoneal cavity, along a pressure gradient, thus
      normalising ICP.

In patients where hydrocephalus is associated with raised ICP (as in this
case) shunting is indicated. In patients where there is no evidence of
raised ICP, shunting should not be performed and the patient should be
managed conservatively with regular follow-up.

2 a Neurogenic shock
   b High thoracic injury
      Cervical spine injury
      Brain injury
   c Compromise of the descending sympathetic pathways in the spinal
      cord.
   d There is a loss of vasomotor tone and sympathetic innervation to
      the heart.
      This results in vasodilatation and pooling of blood in the
      extremities, and this therefore leads to hypotension and an effective
      reduction in circulating volume.
      There is no reflex tachycardia in response to this reduction in
      venous return to the heart, as sympathetic innervation to the heart
      is lost.

e   Neurogenic shock is characterised by a lack of blood pressure response to fluid resuscitation, although a response is seen to vasopressor therapy, secondary to an increase in peripheral vascular tone.

f   Spinal shock is characterised by flaccidity and loss of reflexes following spinal cord injury.

Neurogenic shock is a type of distributive shock. The mainstay of treatment in a patient in which neurogenic shock is suspected is adequate fluid resuscitation. The introduction of vasoactive agents such as noradrenaline, is then utilised to restore systemic vascular resistance.

3 a   Central cord syndrome

b   Hyperextension of the cervical spine

c   Osteophyte/intervertebral disc anteriorly, ligamentum flavum posteriorly.

d   Cervical spondylosis and osteoarthritis

e   Anterior cord syndrome is characterised by severe injury to the majority of the spinal cord.
It commonly occurs after compression fracture of a vertebral body. There is compromise of the corticospinal and spinothalamic tracts leading to a loss of power and reduction in temperature and pain sensation below the level of the lesion. There is sparing of the dorsal column, leading to sparing of proprioception and deep pressure sensation.
In central cord syndrome, there is flaccid weakness of the upper limbs but motor and sensory supply to the lower limbs are preserved as they are located more peripherally in the cord.

f   Anterior spinal artery

Central cord syndrome is characterised by greater impairment of neurological function in the upper limbs as compared to the lower limbs. Bladder dysfunction is common and the patient may present in urinary retention. Depending upon the degree of instability in the cervical spine, treatment may be surgical or conservative.

4 a   Intra-cerebral SOL

b   This states that the cranium behaves like a fixed volume box. The contents of the box (blood, brain and cerebrospinal fluid) are not compressible. As the box is a fixed volume, an increase in one of its constituents, in this case brain tissue secondary to a SOL, will lead to an increase in pressure within the cranium (ICP).

c One of the manifestations of raised ICP that can be detected on physical examination is papilloedema. This can be present with or without obstruction to the normal flow and absorption of CSF. Seizure activity resulting from an SOL is due to mass effect, causing compression of motor pathways within the brain and brainstem. Papilloedema is caused by raised ICP resulting from the SOL (as per the Monro-Kelly doctrine). Each optic nerve is encased in a sheath which is continuous with the pia, arachnoid and dura mater and as such increased ICP is transmitted through to the optic nerve. Fibres of the optic disc then become engorged as a result, represented as papilloedema.

d Lumbar puncture in this patient, without prior investigation, is absolutely contraindicated due to the possibility of brainstem herniation.

e CT brain

Features suggestive of an intracranial neoplasm are changes in personality, lethargy, severe headache and new onset epilepsy. Any of these presenting symptoms, in combination with judicious clinical assessment, justifies imaging in the form of a CT scan.

5 a SAH

b Arteriovenous malformation
Ruptured cerebral aneurysm
Cocaine abuse
Sickle cell disease
Traumatic brain injury

c Aberrant blood within the CSF may lead to irritation of the meninges. The patient may therefore present with symptoms of meningism, including neck stiffness, and photophobia, and therefore it is important to exclude bacterial/viral meningitis.

d CT head in the first instance. If this was inconclusive, a lumbar puncture may be performed, looking for xanthochromia.

e Middle cerebral artery
Posterior inferior cerebellar artery

The initial management of SAH, as with all medical emergencies, is the ABCDE approach. Initial therapy should be focused on the control of blood pressure and fluid and electrolyte balance. The use of nimodipine has been shown to reduce spasm of the intracerebral vessels and limit the size of any potential ischaemic area.

6 a Extradural haematoma

   b The area of the skull commonly fractured is the pterion, at the temperoparietal junction. This is the weakest part of the skull vault. The vessel underlying this area is the middle meningeal artery.

   c A convex, high attenuation area in the temperoparietal region. There may be compression of the ipsilateral lateral ventricle and dilatation of the contralateral lateral ventricle due to compression of the foramen of Munro.

   d Fixed and dilated ipsilateral pupil due to compression of the oculomotor nerve (CN III).
   The oculomotor nerve provides parasympathetic fibres, originating in the Edinger–Westphal nucleus, to the sphincter papillae. Therefore, compromise of the oculomotor nerve will lead to loss of papillary constriction.

   e Using the ABCDE approach to management, it should be recognised at the earliest opportunity that this patient has a GCS <8 and therefore by definition has an unsafe airway. Urgent anaesthetic review should be requested with a view to intubation and ventilation. Following urgent CT brain, the patient should proceed to emergency craniotomy and evacuation of haematoma.

Extradural haematoma commonly occurs following a history of trauma. It is commonly referred to as the 'talk and die' scenario, as a period of lucidity is followed by a rapid deterioration in conscious level. The key to a good outcome is early diagnosis and surgical evacuation.

7 a Chronic subdural haematoma

   b Subdural haemorrhage may be acute or chronic. Fresh blood appears white (hyperdense) on a CT scan, whereas old blood will appear darker in comparison to the cerebral tissue (hypodense).

   c A chronic subdural haematoma may occur after minor trauma. They commonly occur in at-risk patient groups, such as the elderly and patients with a history of alcohol excess, secondary to cerebral atrophy leading to an increase in tension within bridging veins. This makes the bridging veins more susceptible to shearing forces and hence only minor forces can lead to vessel rupture.

   d Altered level of consciousness (decreased GCS)
   Right-sided hemiparesis (contralateral to side of haematoma)
   Fixed and dilated left pupil (secondary to oculomotor nerve compression)
   Papilloedema (secondary to raised ICP)

   e Burr-hole evacuation

Acute subdural haematomas that are small, causing no midline shift or neurological signs may be treated conservatively with regular neurological observations. Chronic subdural haematomas that cause no significant neurological deficits may also be treated conservatively.

If the haematoma requires evacuation then two possible options exist; burr hole evacuation or craniotomy.

8 a Cerebral abscess
   b CT brain with IV contrast
   c No, due to the risk of tentorial herniation
   d Signs of raised ICP
      Hemiplegia
      Loss of sensation
      Cranial nerve palsy
   e Organisms: staphylococcus aureus, haemophilus influenzae
      Management plan – IV fluids and resuscitation, anaesthetic review in view of on-going tonic-clonic seizure activity, and possible need for intubation and ventilation, broad spectrum IV antibiotic therapy initially, followed by specific antibiotic therapy after culture of aspiration known.

A brain abscess is a SOL which produces focal neurological signs. Immunocompromised patients are particularly at risk. Aspiration of the abscess, in order to obtain culture and sensitivity should be performed using 3D imaging.

9 a Pituitary adenoma
      CT or MRI brain
   b Acromegaly
   c Upper quadrantic bitemporal hemianopia secondary to compression of the lower decussating fibres in the optic chiasm.
   d Depression of the papillary reflexes due to destruction of the optic axons which mediate the afferent arc of the papillary light reflex.
   e Prolactin
      TSH
      ACTH
      FSH
      LH

Pituitary adenomas often cause compression of the optic chiasm. They may secrete prolactin, TSH, ACTH, FSH, LH, or growth hormone, and therefore present in a variety of ways. Bromocriptine, radiotherapy and endoscopic removal are the treatment options in this case.

10 a Brown–Sequard syndrome
  b Hemisection of the cord results in paralysis on the affected side inferior to the lesion, accompanied by loss of fine touch discrimination and position sense (proprioception).
    The spinothalamic tract carries fibres which decussate at a lower level, leading to the loss of temperature and pain sensation on the opposite side.
  c Motor – pyramidal tract
    Proprioception/touch – posterior column
  d Inflammatory processes of the CNS (multiple sclerosis)
    Infection (TB)
    Spinal cord ischaemia
  e MRI spine

Brown-Sequard syndrome is characterised by ipsilateral hemiplegia and loss of contralateral pain and temperature sensation. It may progress to complete paralysis or it may resolve completely, depending on the severity and cause of the initial spinal cord insult.

EMQs

1	**A**	10	**E**	19	**A**
2	**H**	11	**I**	20	**B**
3	**I**	12	**E**	21	**F**
4	**D**	13	**J**	22	**G**
5	**E**	14	**F**	23	**A**
6	**D**	15	**H**	24	**I**
7	**G**	16	**D**	25	**E**
8	**C**	17	**F**		
9	**F**	18	**E**		

MCQs

1 d – The GCS assesses verbal, motor and eye opening responses.
2 d – Classical presentation of a SAH is one of severe headache, without relief from analgesia. SAH may occur spontaneously or as a result of trauma. The patient may present with signs of meningism.
3 e – Forced hyperextension of the neck can lead to fracture of the posterior vertebral column, leading to injury of the posterior columns of the spinal cord. This, therefore, causes impairment of joint position sense (proprioception).

4   d – Base of skull fractures present with subconjunctival haemorrhages, periorbital haematoma and bruising around the mastoid process (Battle's Sign). If the fracture extends into the middle cranial fossa the patient may present with CSF otorrhoea/rhinorrea and facial nerve palsy. Anosmia will occur if there is associated injury to the cribriform plate.

5   c – Cerebral contusions occur as a consequence of trauma. They represent bruising on the under-surface of the brain, most commonly in the temporal and frontal regions. Contusions may lead to an increase in ICP due to associated cerebral oedema.

6   b – IIIrd nerve palsy gives rise to ptosis, secondary to paralysis of levator palpabrae superioris, and a fixed and dilated pupil, secondary to paralysis of constrictor papillae. The eye is 'down and out' due to paralysis of all extraocular muscles except lateral rectus and superior oblique.

7   d – Acute subdural haematoma is represented by a hyperdense, concave area on CT brain. If there is associated midline shift and GCS deterioration, the patient should proceed to urgent burr hole evacuation.

8   c – Peak incidence of astrocytoma is early middle age, whilst the peak incidence of medulloblastoma is in childhood. Glioblastoma multiforme is the most malignant form of cerebral tumour. Acoustic neuroma commonly presents with sensorineural deafness and tinnitus.

9   b – The spread of infection from the ethmoidal air sinus, via the ophthalmic vein, to the cavernous sinus may result in cavernous sinus thrombosis. Paralysis of eye movements occurs because of impingement on CN III, IV and VI.

10   a – Flaccid areflexia and a paradoxical breathing pattern point towards cervical cord transection. Initial examination findings that would further support this diagnosis are priapism and a loss of anal tone on digital rectal examination.